Updates in Clinical Dermatology

Updates in Clinical Dermatology aims to promote the rapid and efficient transfer of medical research into clinical practice. It is published in four volumes per year. Covering new developments and innovations in all fields of clinical dermatology, it provides the clinician with a review and summary of recent research and its implications for clinical practice. Each volume is focused on a clinically relevant topic and explains how research results impact diagnostics, treatment options and procedures as well as patient management. The reader-friendly volumes are highly structured with core messages, summaries, tables, diagrams and illustrations and are written by internationally well-known experts in the field. A volume editor supervises the authors in his/her field of expertise in order to ensure that each volume provides cutting-edge information most relevant and useful for clinical dermatologists. Contributions to the series are peer reviewed by an editorial board.

Esraa M. AlEdani • Howard Maibach
Editors

Mesotherapy and Its Medical Applications

Springer

Editors
Esraa M. AlEdani
Basra Medical College
Basrah, Iraq

Howard Maibach
University of California, San Francisco
San Francisco, CA, USA

ISSN 2523-8884 ISSN 2523-8892 (electronic)
Updates in Clinical Dermatology
ISBN 978-3-031-76069-3 ISBN 978-3-031-76070-9 (eBook)
https://doi.org/10.1007/978-3-031-76070-9

This Springer imprint is published by the registered company Springer Nature Switzerland AG
The registered company address is: Gewerbestrasse 11, 6330 Cham, Switzerland

Preface

Mesotherapy, a cosmetic procedure that has advanced significantly since its inception, is at the intersection of medical innovation and cosmetic dermatology. This collection of essays delves deeply into the history, mechanics, and uses of mesotherapy, with a special emphasis on its function in dermatological problems. The chapters are designed to provide both core information and in-depth insights into the numerous dermatological disorders where mesotherapy has shown promise.

The first chapter delves into the history and fundamental concepts of mesotherapy, providing a thorough explanation of the procedures and classifications that define this minimally invasive approach. It builds the framework for understanding how mesotherapy operates at the cellular level and its ability to provide tailored therapeutic advantages. In contrast, the second chapter discusses the role of mesotherapy in skin rejuvenation and its significant role in aging and youth.

Chapter 3 expands on this basis by investigating the use of mesotherapy to treat particular dermatological disorders, such as acne, melasma, rosacea, and androgenetic alopecia. Through a review of current research and clinical trials, this chapter demonstrates the usefulness of mesotherapy in these aspects, presenting it as a flexible tool in the dermatologist's field. In contrast, Chap. 4 explores the role of dermatology in nondermatological diseases and how these clinical trials and studies show mesotherapy as a promising alternative for managing pain, musculoskeletal system, etc.

Chapter 5 elaborates on the unexpected side effects that skin may experience as a result of mesotherapy. In contrast, Chap. 6 focuses on the role of mesotherapy in the market, highlighting how it is often used as a lucrative business to promise treatments for acne or pigmentation.

As the field of mesotherapy continues to expand, these chapters seek to add to the core information supporting its safe and successful usage. Whether you are a practitioner or new to the topic, this compilation provides essential insights that will help you better understand and apply mesotherapy in clinical practice.

Basrah, Iraq — Esraa M. AlEdani
San Francisco, CA, USA — Howard Maibach

Contents

Chapter 1
Mesotherapy Background, Mechanisms, Techniques and Classification

Esraa M. AlEdani

1.1 Overview

Mesotherapy is a noninvasive skin rejuvenation procedure. Mesotherapy is a procedure that involves multiple intradermic injections or injections of a mixture of compounds containing bioactive substances, mucopolysaccharides, prescribed drugs, plant extracts, medical aid agents, and vitamins in minute doses and is administered with incredibly fine-gauge needles to treat native medical and cosmetic conditions. The mechanism of action of mesotherapy is that solutions injected into the germ layer remain within the space for a longer period than they would be disseminated by deeper injection, as they are added bit by the final circulation. The needle penetration depth must not exceed four metric linear units. Mesotherapy is used to treat a variety of local medical and cosmetic issues, including loss of skin tone, loss of radiance, skin aging, superficial wrinkles, and hair loss.

The term "meso" means "middle" and refers to the injection method (into the middle layer of skin or "intradermotherapy") as well as the average amount of drug administered (dose in between allopathy and homeopathy). Mesotherapy does not refer to a specific treatment; rather, it denotes a mechanism of medication administration. Mesotherapy is performed on structures derived from the mesoderm rather than the mesoderm itself, as the latter ceases to exist beyond the embryonic stage of human development. It has been proposed that when medications are administered via mesotherapy, the skin serves as a natural time-release mechanism. Other benefits claimed for mesotherapy include low-cost equipment, relatively little training required for providers, immediate and undiluted delivery of drugs to the target area, much lower drug dosage requirements, faster achievement of benefits, minimal invasiveness and thus attendant pain, and no need for hospitalization.

E. M. AlEdani (✉)
Basra Medical College, Basrah, Iraq

E. M. AlEdani, H. Maibach (eds.), *Mesotherapy and Its Medical Applications*, Updates in Clinical Dermatology, https://doi.org/10.1007/978-3-031-76070-9_1

The scientific basis for this procedure is based on preclinical research showing that a medication injected at small dosages into the surface layer of the skin travels slowly to the underlying tissues and stays longer than systemic delivery. In fact, compared with intramuscular administration, greater amounts of intradermally injected medication have been discovered in the skin, muscles, and joints underneath the infiltration site. One of the primary benefits of mesotherapy is the medication-sparing effect compared with the deeper route of delivery.

Furthermore, the dose-saving effect has been thoroughly shown in the context of immunoprophylaxis via intradermal methods. Furthermore, it has been postulated that the microdamage caused by the needle, as well as the chemical–physical interactions caused by the liquid infiltrating into the dermis, might cause dermal responses capable of amplifying the impact of the medication injected into the dermis. These intradermal processes, known as mesodermal modulation, are theories that must be tested experimentally.

1.2 Background

Injections into the skin for medicinal purposes have a long history, starting with Hippocrates (400 B.C.), who used a topical application of cactus for shoulder discomfort; in Chinese medicine, acupuncture has been used by the Chinese for 2000 years, and the injection of drugs has been used since the introduction of the hollow needle in the nineteenth century. More recently, in 1847, Karl Baunscheidt became convinced that a medicine might act even if it was just superficially injected and underwent cutaneous injection at a depth of two millimeters. Alexander Wood (a Scottish physician) injected the first dosage of dermic morphine to relieve pain in a variety of painful conditions in 1853. Bartolomeo Guala initiated systematic hypodermic therapy in a hospital in 1860, and Gaetano Primavera in Naples conducted the first experiment to determine the degree of medication absorption in the urine following hypodermic delivery in 1867. The London Medical Society wrote in the same year about hypodermic injections, citing "the speed, intensity, and safety of the action, the production of a given effect with a lower dose of the other administrations, the certainty of the effects, the ease of application, the absence of certain disagreeable actions of other drugs". Doctors injected distilled water into the dermis to mitigate arthritic pain during the Franco-Prussian War in 1870. In 1885, William Halsted reported that intradermal injection of sterile water causes local anesthesia. Pietro Orlandini, a Venetian doctor, recommended dermal punctures for the treatment of specific kinds of localized pain in 1894, whereas George D. Gammon and Isaac Starr described the analgesic efficacy of sterile water injection into the skin in 1941.

In 1958, Michel Pistor used the term "mesotherapy" to describe drug injection in the skin. Sergio Maggiori developed the term "local intradermal therapy" (LIT) in 2004, after reviewing preclinical and clinical data, to stress that superficial inoculation allowed for clinical improvement with a lower drug dosage. In 1945, Pistor began injecting small amounts of medication into the mesoderm as a treatment for deafness. His first professional paper on mesotherapy was published in 1952. In 1987, mesotherapy was recognized as a medical specialty by the French Academy of Medicine. In 1975, the Italian Society of Mesotherapy began to legitimize mesotherapy with preclinical research to determine the pharmacokinetics of active substances injected intradermally. Numerous clinical trials have been performed to confirm the effectiveness and tolerance of localized paint in a variety of clinical situations.

The procedure has since been used to treat some pain syndromes, arthritis, vascular and lymphatic disorders, alopecia, and bone and joint disorders. The procedure was subsequently adapted for cosmetic purposes to contour the body, remove cellulite, and rejuvenate the skin. This technique, which has been used for decades in Europe and South America, has recently become popular in the United States. Mesotherapy is promoted as a noninvasive, painless, and safer alternative to liposuction.

To date, LIT is among the most well-known and commonly used microinvasive methods in many areas of the world for treating various local clinical problems. Over the past few years, patients have frequently asked, "How does mesotherapy work?" to address this matter.

1.3 Mesotherapy Component

Mesotherapy involves the injection of drugs, reagents, and plant extracts into the adipose and connective tissue layers under the skin. Injectables include a variety of compounds used to open blood vessels, nonsteroidal anti-inflammatory drugs, enzymes, nutrients, antibiotics, and hormones. For mesotherapy, two key compounds, the fundamental constituents of Lipostabil, are used: phosphatidylcholine (PC) and deoxycholic acid. Most mesotherapy clinics and linked websites appear to employ Lipostabil or a clone, either alone or in conjunction with additional substances. Mesotherapy drugs differ from doctor to doctor, as do the number and frequency of injections (there is no standardization of dosing).

As a result, no protocol or treatment algorithm is available to enable physicians to anticipate how much tissue or fat will be "dissolved" with a certain solution, in a set amount, and injected at a specified subcutaneous tissue depth.

1.3.1 Phosphatidylcholine

A glycerol backbone is connected to three attached groups: two long-chain fatty acids and choline. When PC is consumed, the majority of it is degraded into choline, glycerol-free fatty acids, and phosphate groups rather than being absorbed intact into cellular membranes. When discussing mesotherapy, it is unclear what happens to PC when it is injected into the skin in large quantities. When injected into an aqueous environment, PC can exist in three distinct chemical forms, according to lipidologists.

Phosphatidylcholine, at low molar concentrations, produces lipid bilayers, a chemical arrangement comparable to that of cell membranes. Under agitation, PC molecules can form discrete vesicle structures with an aqueous-containing internal core. Micelles with organic soluble cores develop at greater concentrations (4×10^{-10} M), which are known as critical micelle concentrations (CMCs). This is significant because triglycerides released from ruptured fat cells cannot be carried by a PC bilayer or a PC vesicle, but a PC micelle can solubilize and transport triglycerides and free fatty acids. If Lipostabil is injected at 90% (w/v), PC will exist mostly as a micelle. However, mesotherapists employ different solutions, and the chemical form(s) involved remain unknown.

The interactions of phosphatidylcholine with cell membranes have been studied. Phosphatidylcholine improved cholesterol solubility. Furthermore, PC-rich lipoproteins are found outside of subcutaneous adipocytes as high-density lipoproteins (HDLs), which act as transporters of excess cholesterol from extrahepatic cells to the liver.

Intracellular cholesteryl esters can be mobilized in the context of mesotherapy to generate free cholesterol, which is subsequently distributed via plasma membranes and transported by HDL. Triglycerides, as well as cholesteryl esters, may be hydrolyzed to glycerol and free fatty acids during this process. Free fatty acids diffuse across the membrane and are carried by albumin. As a result, there is a metabolic route for reducing adipocyte fat levels that does not involve necrosis and requires PC-rich particles. HDL cholesterol levels increased when doses ranging from 1.5 g once a day to 3.5 g three times daily were used in many clinical trials assessing Lipostabil.

1.3.2 Deoxycholic Acid

Deoxycholic acid is the second most important component of Lipostabil. High amounts of deoxycholate, a bile salt, are known to be hazardous to the cutaneous and pulmonary systems. Deoxycholate can occur in two forms, according to chemists. The first is a monomer (CMC = 5×10^{-3} M), and the second is a micelle. If the deoxycholate level claimed in Lipostabil is used, CMC will be insufficient (2.0 g/L vs. CMC of 2.1 g/L) to fulfill the micelle status, and deoxycholate will exist mostly as a monomer if injected alone. However, if PC is injected, mixed micelles or micelles containing both components should be present, and excess deoxycholate should be present in the form of monomers. A 3-phase chart can be used to forecast various physical forms. With low cholesterol concentrations in the extracellular environment, different phases can occur, including micelles, vesicles, and crystals (which can harm cells). With the existing formulations, it is only possible to guess which physical shape is offered to adipocytes.

It would seem natural that a micellar presentation format may facilitate modest fat mobilization from cells, but vesicle presentation with excess monomers of deoxycholate may be related to enhanced cellular necrosis. Cellular damage is connected with crystal formation. The FDA raised major concerns and unsolved issues on the basis of these several conceivable permutations of physical forms and tissue reactions (mobilization, necrosis, and unknown consequences) following injection with recognized dietary reagents.

1.3.3 Peptides

Acetyldecapeptide-3 works to minimize and prevent wrinkles by actively creating new skin cells.

- **Decapeptide-4**: for wound healing and antiaging
- **Copper tripeptide-1**: improves blood circulation and revitalizes the skin.
- **Oligopeptide-24**: reduces scars on the skin by creating new skin cells.
- **Tripeptide-6** moistens dry skin and maintains an optimal moisture balance

Others include pentapeptide, L-carnitine, and liquorice. Biopeptides are a significant component of mesolift, mesoglow, mesocellulite, mesohair, and mesosculpting because of the features listed above.

1.3.4 Growth Factors and Stem Cells

Thymosin TB-4, a growth factor, is injected into the mesoderm of the scalp, i.e., directly into hair follicles, as part of scalp mesotherapy. TB-4 promotes hair follicle development by increasing circulation, activating stem cells, and revitalizing hair follicles. Because of their proliferative ability, stem cells derived from bone marrow are a significant component of whitening serum and wrinkling solutions. Stem cells are currently widely used in whitening treatments.

1.3.5 Platelet-Rich Plasma

For scalp mesotherapy, a tiny amount of blood is collected from the patient and quickly centrifuged, and the platelet concentrate is injected intradermally into the scalp. Platelet growth factors and healing proteins enhance circulation to hair follicles, causing hair follicle development and, as a result, hair growth.

Growth factors such as platelet-derived growth factor, transforming growth factor, and vascular endothelial growth factor released from platelet alfa granules increase fibroblast proliferation and dermal fibroblast production of procollagen type 1 carboxy peptide, improving skin structural integrity.

Platelet-rich plasma (PRP) can be employed in photoaged and aged skin because of this feature. PRP also stimulates the development of matrix metalloproteinases, which breakdown and eliminate collagen fragments that interfere with the synthesis of new collagen in aged skin. As a result, PRP aids in skin remodeling.

However, further research is needed to confirm the safety of PRP as a component of mesotherapy. Typically, maintenance therapy is performed once every 4–6 months for a year and then once a year, depending on the patient's reaction.

1.4 Mechanism of Mesotherapy

Once the medicine is administered by mesotherapy, the skin serves as a natural time-release mechanism. The mechanism of action of mesotherapy is that solutions injected intracutaneously stay inside the area for much longer than if they are disseminated by deeper injection. These treatments involve vitamins, trace components, enzymes, antioxidants, organic compounds, and other active ingredients that improve skin quality. These ingredients, when absorbed by the skin, promote albuminoid and elastin formation, rebuild the inner structure of the skin, smooth wrinkles, restore skin tone and snap, and restore a healthy glowing appearance. The major effect of mesotherapy is a regenerated, lower-classman face, as well as a second type of massage, which increases skin firmness and allows for reasonable stretching.

Even though mesotherapy has been routinely utilized in Europe for years to cure cellulite, the underlying mechanism remains unclear. To the best of our knowledge, no clinical scientific research supporting mesotherapy has been published in the literature. It is hypothesized that it begins to increase blood and lymphatic flow in the mesoderm. This causes fat cells to shrink, causing them to disintegrate and be expelled. The issue is the scarcity of randomized, double-blind trials conducted under institutional review board-approved protocols to assure patient safety. The FDA has not authorized the subcutaneous administration of the medications routinely used in mesotherapy. According to the available data, these drugs have the potential to produce immediate or delayed allergic responses, including urticaria pigmentosa at the injection sites.

1.5 Indication

Mesotherapy, such as corticosteroids, has a wide range of uses, particularly in cosmetic dermatology. However, only the most recent and commonly utilized indications in dermatology, as well as the medications employed in them, are described here.

1. Body cellulite, Lipodissolve, and body contouring (ineffective)
2. Skin renewal/glow, lift, and pigmentation
3. androgenetic alopecia, hair telogen effluvium

1.6 Techniques

Several mesotherapy procedures differ according to the needle gauge and length, the injected substances or resolution, the depth of needle penetration, and the portions of the injected layer. Intraepidermic (IED), nappage, purpose-by-purpose (PPP), mesoperfusion, and hypodermic methods are a few typical procedures in mesotherapy.

1.6.1 Intraepidermal (IED)

Perrin was the first to define this technique in 1989. It is the most obvious of the remaining approaches. When this method is performed correctly, the needle does not enter the basal layer. A 13 mm, 27–30 gauge needle is positioned at the closest angle of the skin. Once the needle's bevel is pointed away from the skin, the syringe is dragged across the skin with gradual, lightweight positive pressure.

1.6.2 Nappage

First defined by Sauce and Ravily, it is an extra surface technique that requires practice to perfect. During this procedure, a 4 mm needle is used with the syringe command at a 40–45 degree angle to the skin. The depth of penetration is merely 0.5–2 mm, and a drop of solution is injected at each location at a distance of 0.25–0.5 cm via mild, steady positive pressure on the plunger. Nappage is the least comfortable procedure disclosed by the patient.

1.6.3 Point-By-Point (PPP)

The UN agency that discovered the point-by-point approach was Dr. Pistor. The operation is rather simple to carry out. A syringe holding approximately 0.02 cc to 0.05 cc of solution is injected sheer at 4 mm, 6 mm, or 12 mm of total depth. These injections are usually delivered at a distance of 1–2 cm.

1.6.4 Meso Perfusion

The needle used in the Mesoperfusion method is known as a Lebel needle, and its bevel is four millimeters long. Its length is determined by the method employed, which ranges from 4–15 mm tiny needles (27–30 gauge).

1.6.5 Papule Formation

The medications are injected between 2 and 4 mm from the dermoepidermal junction, causing tiny papules to form. Typically, it is used to treat wrinkles, alopecia, and mesobotox.

1.6.6 Point by Point

It involves injecting 0.02–0.05 mL of medication solution perpendicular to the skin (4 mm deep) approximately 1–2 cm apart. It is mostly used to burn fat.

1.6.7 Epidermal

It is the most superficial (1 mm deep) of all the procedures since the skin's basal layer is not pierced. The needle is inserted and pulled along with the plunger under modest, positive pressure. It is applied in a grid pattern at 1 cm intervals throughout the afflicted region.

1.7 No Needle Mesotherapy NNM

It is a revolutionary mesotherapy modification that allows both ionized and neutral medicines to be delivered into the dermis and subcutaneous tissue. The chosen spot is initially pretreated with dual-wavelength laser light and then contains four components:

(a) **Electroporation**: Electric waves of three distinct frequencies result in electrophoresis of the skin, ranging in size from 40 to 250 μm. The desired compounds are then made to pass through these pores via electrorepulsion. However, because of their form, neutral substances can also flow through pores.
(b) **Active current**: This current enhances vascularity and guarantees that an adequate product reaches the desired location.

(c) **Hydrophoresis**: the penetration of water-soluble compounds into the skin.
(d) **Cryophoresis**: the freezing of chemicals in skin cells.

No needle mesotherapy (NNM) is primarily used to treat cellulite, but it is also useful for skin rejuvenation, hyperpigmentation from photoaging, wrinkle reduction, pore reduction, and skin lifting tightness. Compared with those of mesotherapy, the advantages of NNM include (a) that it is painless; (b) that it does not cause bruising, erythema, or swelling; (c) that materials can permeate to deeper levels; (d) that it can cause immediate/rapid reactions; and (d) that it is cost efficient.

1.8 Classification

A solution typically comprises a principal/major component (P) with strong effectiveness data and complementary/minor compounds (C). The constituents of any solution should be water soluble, isotonic, or nonallergenic. A solution often consists of a carrier solution (such as procaine, lidocaine, or NaCl) as well as vitamins, vasoactive agents, and herbal medicines, among other compounds, depending on the condition being treated. The mesosolution or mesococktail is chosen on the basis of the indication.

1.8.1 Mesolift/Biorejuvenation

"Mesolift"is a combination of multivitamins, plant stem cells, antioxidants, and noncross-linked, high-viscosity hyaluronic acid that hydrates the skin and results in a smoother and firmer appearance.

The following are some of the most popular agents used in biorevitalization solutions:

1.8.1.1 Hyaluronic Acid (HA))

The appeal of HA as a mesotherapy agent arises from its large molecular size and difficulty in passing through the skin barrier and reaching the dermis. Because of its capacity to bind water molecules, HA serves a vital function in the hydration of the extracellular space. It also generates physiological conditions in the extracellular matrix for dermal cell proliferation, migration, and organization.

There is substantial evidence to support the clinical and histological effectiveness of HA-based mesotherapy in increasing dermal collagen fiber density via fibroblast activation, consequently enhancing skin hydration, firmness, and viscoelastic characteristics. HA combines with snake tripeptide or Synake [(2S)-beta-alanyl-L-prolyl-2,4-diamino-N (phenylmethyl)butanamide acetate], which blocks neurotransmission in the nicotinic acetylcholine receptor, which helps decrease the number of fine lines and imparts a firmer feel (Meso-cheek lift).

In addition, a unique formulation of 27 mg of noncrosslinked, supersonically modified low-molecular-weight HA was mixed with copper tripeptide and keratinocyte growth factor, fibroblast growth factor, insulin-like growth factor, and epidermal growth factor. The low molecular weight of the formulation not only penetrates deep into the dermis but also works as a carrier for growth. In various formulations, different concentrations of HA are mixed with vitamins, plant stem cells, and other substances. In our opinion, HA works best when paired with a microneedling device for younger people with dehydrated skin or a radiofrequency microneedling device for elderly people with inelastic and dehydrated skin.

Depending on the clinical picture, HA mesotherapy is also commonly used for areas such as the dorsal hand, neck, and neck, where it may be combined with other modalities such as soft tissue fillers, the mesobotox technique, threads, fractional resurfacing, and/or the quasilong pulse mode of the Q-switched Nd YAG laser.

1.8.1.2 Dimethylaminoethanol (DMAE)

DMAE is a precursor of phosphatidylcholine (PPC), which transforms choline into acetylcholine (Ach) and other phospholipids. As a result, muscular contraction occurs, resulting in muscle stiffness (mostly in the lower face). DMAE also promotes the formation of proteoglycans. It can be coupled with the following items:

- **Silicium**—This trace element interacts with collagen and elastin fibers, enhancing proteoglycans in the skin. They aid in fighting muscular tiredness and enhance wound healing.
- **Dipeptide Carnosine**—A histidine derivative, commonly known as the Meso eye lift, is believed to increase skin firmness.

1.8.1.3 Peptides

Peptides are skin rejuvenation agents. These biopeptides play a vital role in mesolift, mesoglow, mesocellulose, mesohair, and mesosculpting.

(a) **Decapeptide-4** has antiaging and wound-healing properties.
(b) **Copper tripeptide-1**: Improving skin blood circulation
(c) **Oligopeptide-24:** Aids in collagen rebuilding
(d) **Tripeptide-6:** Hydrates dry skin and maintains it at its optimal moisture level.

1.8.2 Mesoglow

Glutathione and ascorbic acid are the major constituents, as are kojic acid, glycolic acid, pyruvic acid, azelaic acid, and plant extracts, which can brighten and reduce superficial pigmentary abnormalities. The technique is frequently performed weekly or biweekly for 4–6 sessions. For the best results, Mesoglow can be combined with medical therapy, such as skin lightening agents or cosmeceuticals, as well as alternating sessions of Q-switched Nd:YAG toning or shallow-to-medium-depth chemical peels.

1.8.3 Mesobotox

Mesobotox or Microbotox involves the delivery of botulinum toxin to superficial, uniformly sized droplets in the dermis for optimum results. The amount or dilution of botulinum toxin is critical since too little botulinum toxin will result in unsatisfactory results and a dissatisfied patient, whereas too much botulinum toxin will result in a large droplet size that will be administered in the wrong plane, resulting in unpleasant effects. Microbotox operates on the superficial layer of facial muscles that are linked to the dermal undersurface, preserving the function of the deeper muscle fibers and delivering a natural look. Fine lines and wrinkles are decreased by weakening the facial muscles rather than completely paralyzing them. Furthermore, microbotox causes bulk atrophy of sweat and sebaceous glands, which improves skin texture and shines. Mesobotox has recently been utilized to relax muscle fibers in the scalp, resulting in dilatation of the blood vessels in the scalp area and improved delivery of nutrients to hair follicles. Microbotox can be used for the following conditions, although it is most successful in treating rhytids of the neck and lower face.

1.8.4 Meso-Cellulite

All are principal agents:

- L-carnitine
- Aminophylline
- Pentoxiphylline
- DMAE
- Vitamin C
- Procaine

1.8.5 Mesostretch

All are principal agents:

- Silorgamine = silorg + DMAE or
- Idebe = idebenone + DMAE or
- Centella asiatica, fibronectin, vegetal proteins.

1.8.6 Localized Lipodissolve/Injection Lipolysis (Chin Jowls, Double Chin, Eye Pad Fats)

Deoxycholate and phosphatidyl vitamin B (PC) are the most often utilized fat-dissolving agents. Phosphatidyi is an inhibitor made from soybean phospholipids. At a dosage of 250 mg, the depth of injection for injection lipolysis and localized fat deposition varies from half a dozen mm to twelve millimeters. When phosphatidyl acid enters adipocyte cells, it breaks down fat cells, which are then expelled by the urinary organ system via the bloodstream. It (b) promotes lipolysis by activating receptors and inhibiting a pair of adipocyte membrane receptors. (c) It also induces inflammatory cytokine-mediated gangrene and adipocyte organic processes.

When the inflammation that promotes retraction of the unsearled tissues diminishes, new scleroprotein is produced.

1.8.7 Hair Mesotherapy

The use of mesos for hair loss promises to increase hair quality, hydration, anagen phase prolongation, microcirculation, and nutrient delivery and to block 5-alpha reductase. Despite a dearth of controlled published research on mesotherapy in hair diseases, injections of minoxidil, finasteride, dutasteride, saw palmetto, biotin, panthenol, hyaluronic acid, taurine, and multivitamins are used to treat alopecia.

Mesohair treatment is not indicated for patients suffering from autoimmune diseases such as alopecia areata, frontal fibrosing alopecia, and/or scarring alopecia. In addition to regular medical therapy, mesotherapy for hair loss may be supplemented with low-level laser light therapy (LLLT), platelet-rich plasma (PRP), and/or recombinant human growth factors in the same or different sessions for more effective results.

Further Reading

1. Brown SA. The science of mesotherapy: chemical anarchy. Aesthet Surg J. 2006;26(1):95–8. https://doi.org/10.1016/j.asj.2005.12.003.
2. Mammucari M, Maggiori E, Russo D, Giorgio C, Ronconi G, Ferrara PE, Canzona F, Antonaci L, Violo B, Vellucci R, Mediati DR, Migliore A, Massafra U, Bifarini B, Gori F, di Carlo M, Brauneis S, Paolucci T, Rocchi P, Cuguttu A, Di Marzo R, Bomprezzi A, Santini S, Giardini M, Catizzone AR, Troili F, Dorato D, Gallo A, Guglielmo C, Natoli S. Mesotherapy: from historical notes to scientific evidence and future prospects. ScientificWorldJournal. 2020;2020:3542848. PMID: 32577099; PMCID: PMC7305548. https://doi.org/10.1155/2020/3542848.
3. Al Faresi F, Galadari HI. Mesotherapy: myth and reality. Expert Rev Dermatol. 2011;6(2):157–62. https://doi.org/10.1586/edm.11.15.
4. Saluja H, Patil AS, Shah S, Dadhich A, Sachdeva S. Mesotherapy: overview. IP Int J Maxillofac Imaging. 2020;6(2):29–32.
5. Sivagnanam G. Mesotherapy—the French connection. J Pharmacol Pharmacother. 2010;1(1):4–8. PMID: 21808584; PMCID: PMC3142757. https://doi.org/10.4103/0976-500X.64529.
6. da Silva RL, de Oliveira FA, Medeiros RG, Cunha SV, Gouveia GPM. What is the physical-mechanical mechanism of pressurized mesotherapy? Med Hypotheses. 2021;152:110617. Epub 2021 May 28. https://doi.org/10.1016/j.mehy.2021.110617.
7. Mammucari M, Paolucci T, Russo D, Maggiori E, Di Marzo R, Migliore A, Massafra U, Ronconi G, Ferrara PE, Gori F, Bifarini B, Brauneis S, Vellucci R, Mediati RD, Violo B, Natoli S, Pediliggieri C, Di Campli C, Collina MC. A call to action by the Italian Mesotherapy society on scientific research. Drug Des Dev Ther. 2021;15:3041–7. PMID: 34285471; PMCID: PMC8285234. https://doi.org/10.2147/DDDT.S321215.
8. Rohrich RJ. Mesotherapy: what is it? Does it work? Plast Reconstr Surg. 2005;115(5):1425. https://doi.org/10.1097/01.prs.0000162243.34988.90.
9. Rotunda AM. Injectable treatments for adipose tissue: terminology, mechanism, and tissue interaction. Lasers Surg Med. 2009;41(10):714–20. https://doi.org/10.1002/lsm.20807.
10. Konda D, Thappa DM. Mesotherapy: what is new? Indian J Dermatol Venereol Leprol. 2013;79(1):127–34. https://doi.org/10.4103/0378-6323.104689.
11. Business Bliss Consultants FZE. Mesotherapy strategies and techniques. 2018. https://nursinganswers.net/essays/mesotherapy-strategies-techniques-2887.php?vref=1
12. Kutlubay Z, Karakuş Ö. Hair Mesother Hair Ther Transpl. 2012;1:e102. https://doi.org/10.4172/2167-0951.1000e102.
13. Vineetha Reddy N, Jyothi M, Venkatesh P, Hepcy Kalarini D, Prema R. Mesotherapy in face. Int J Res Eng Sci Manag. 2019;2(10):822.
14. Kandhari R, Kaur I, Sharma D. Mesococktails and mesoproducts in aesthetic dermatology. Dermatol Ther. 2020;33(6):e14218. Epub 2020 Sep 10. https://doi.org/10.1111/dth.14218.
15. Rotunda AM, Kolodney MS. Mesotherapy and phosphatidylcholine injections: historical clarification and review. Dermatol Surg. 2006;32(4):465–80. https://doi.org/10.1111/j.1524-4725.2006.32100.x.

Chapter 2
Exploring Mesotherapy, The Rejuvenation Revolution (Or Is It?)

Suhel F. Batarseh and Esraa M. AlEdani

2.1 Overview

Sometimes referred to as biorevitalization or mesolift, biorejuvenation is a word used frequently to describe mesotherapy for skin renewal. This method aims to increase the biosynthesis ability of fibroblasts; stimulate the production of collagen, elastin, and hyaluronisc acid (HA); encourage the restoration of an ideal physiological environment; and increase cell activity. The injection of appropriate, fully absorbable, and entirely biocompatible materials into the superficial dermis can provide the desired result of firm, bright, and moisturized skin.

Because of the natural aging process (chronoaging), the skin changes with time, becoming more atrophic, lax, and wrinkled. These changes might be clinical or histological.

Cumulative environmental deterioration, including smoking tobacco, pollution, and prolonged exposure to UV light (photodamage), can accelerate the aging process.

Mesotherapy is a powerful addition to other noninvasive rejuvenation techniques. Because it revitalizes the skin, fewer operations are needed. In addition to applying sunscreen every day and abstaining from smoking, mesotherapy is an additional antiaging strategy that aids in maintaining firm and bright skin worldwide by shielding it from environmental factors that contribute to aging.

Easy to perform.

- Low pain
- No necessity for skin tests

S. F. Batarseh
Faculty of Medicine, Jordan University of Science and Technology, Ar-Ramtha, Jordan

E. M. AlEdani (✉)
Basra Medical College, Basrah, Iraq

E. M. AlEdani, H. Maibach (eds.), *Mesotherapy and Its Medical Applications*, Updates in Clinical Dermatology, https://doi.org/10.1007/978-3-031-76070-9_2

- Limited side effects
- There was no downtime or recovery time
- Suitable for every skin phototype

There are several items on the market that can be used for biorejuvenation; some are monomers, while others are mixtures of various substances.

- Hyaluronic acid alone (1.35%–3%)
- Hyaluronic acid 0.2%, 1%, or 3% plus other active ingredients
- Polynucleotide macromolecules
- Organic silica
- Autologous cultured fibroblasts
- Growth factors
- Homeopathic products

Recently, injecting a mixture containing just one ingredient has been suggested to be preferable to injecting a cocktail because the side effects from the interactions of the various ingredients should be minimized, and the active ingredients should be more concentrated when they are injected alone.

2.2 Effective Regenerative Components Used in Anti-Aging Mesotherapy

The precise mode of action of mesotherapy is unknown. Fibroblast dysfunction, a decrease in the fibroblast population and the generation of collagen, hyaluronic acid, and other extracellular matrix components, as well as an increase in the fibroblast count, are all consequences of skin aging. Synthesis of the enzymes that breakdown collagen and fibroblasts.

Therefore, the cocktail for mesotherapy should contain micronutrients and biomolecular substances that create a good environment for fibroblast function.

Mesoresolution typically includes complementary/minor compounds and a principal/major component with compelling evidence of effectiveness. The constituents of any solution should be nonallergic, isotonic, or water soluble. Depending on the indication being treated, a mesosolution usually comprises a carrier solution (such as procaine, lidocaine, or NaCl) with vitamins, vasoactive agents, and herbal treatments, among other compounds. On the basis of the indication, either the mesosolution or the mesococktail is selected.

The mesolift is a combination of multivitamins, plant stem cells, antioxidants, and noncross-linked, high-viscosity hyaluronic acid that moistens the skin and results in a smoother, firmer appearance.

One of the common agents of biorevitalization solutions. Owing to its capacity to draw in water molecules, HA is crucial for maintaining the physiological conditions of the extracellular matrix, which support dermal cell migration, proliferation, and organization.

HA, together with copper tripeptide, keratinocyte growth factor, fibroblast growth factor, insulin-like growth factor, and epidermal growth factor, and 27 mg of noncrosslinked, superossified low-molecular-weight HA were mixed together. In addition to penetrating deeply into the dermis, the low molecular weight of the formulation serves as a carrier for growth.

Different formulations mix plant stem cells, vitamins, and other substances with various concentrations of HA, such as 1.30 to 100 mg hyaluronic acid (sodium salt form), five% mannitol, DMAE, procollagen peptide, argireline, leuphasyl, and marine collagen. Silicium is an essential trace element that interacts with collagen and elastin fibers, enriching proteoglycans in the skin. Vitamins B1–B6 (World Dermic, Spain, EU).

Hyaluronic acid (40 mg), vegetal stem cell booster, vitamins A, B5, B3, and B6 (Pluryal Mesoline Refresh, Luxembourg, 5 mL vials × 5) were used.

Additionally, HA combines with Synake, also known as snake tripeptide [(2S)-beta-alanyl-L-prolyl-2,4-diamino-N-(phenylmethyl)butanamide acetate], which is claimed to block nicotinic acetylcholine receptor neurotransmission. This, when combined with hydrating agents, helps reduce fine lines and gives the cheeks a firmer feel.

A recent RCT that evaluated 146 patients revealed that NCTF®135HA®, which is a mesotherapy product that contains a mixture of hyaluronic acid (HA) and various other skin-rejuvenating ingredients. Mesotherapy involves injecting smaller amounts of these substances into the skin to improve its appearance. Was superior to an active control (antiaging cream) in terms of volume reduction and the severity of wrinkles on the neck, décolleté, and crow's feet; the advantages of NCTF®135HA extend beyond the enhancements brought about by antiaging treatments on their own.

Another important agent is **dimethylaminoethanol (DMAE)**, which is a precursor of phosphatidylcholine (PPC), which produces muscular contraction that results in acetylcholine (Ach) (mostly in the lower face). Additionally, DMAE promotes the formation of proteoglycans.

A recent study revealed the benefit of using tranexamic acid (TXA), which is a medication that belongs to the class of antifibrinolytic drugs. It works by inhibiting the breakdown of blood clots, which helps reduce bleeding. Tranexamic acid is often used in medical settings to control or prevent excessive bleeding, especially in situations such as surgeries, dental procedures, and heavy menstrual bleeding.

It has been used to treat pigmented disorders in dermatology for a long time. They concluded that the volume and area of wrinkles are dramatically decreased by tranexamic acid mesotherapy. Transverse agent injections as a mesotherapy appear to be beneficial for improving periorbital wrinkles.

Moreover, recent studies have included 20% L-ascorbic acid in combination with hydrosol. They reported that following microneedle mesotherapy, a formulation containing L-ascorbic acid soluble in hydrolysate significantly enhanced skin elasticity and improved skin conditions.

2.3 Mechanisms by Which Skin Aging Is Reducing

Before discussing the mechanism for reducing skin aging, we need to know what skin aging is.

Aging is biological attrition at the cellular level that results in a decline in reserve capacity and the ability to execute normal tasks, increasing the chance of death. Therefore, aging is the outcome of a genetic clock or programme that is ingrained in each species' genetic makeup. Importantly, the progressive harm to genes and proteins can lead to reduced function and breakdown of homeostasis. This causes the organism to age and die too quickly, which ultimately depends on its ability to heal itself.

Genetics, environmental exposure (UV radiation, xenobiotics, and mechanical stress), hormonal changes, and metabolic processes (production of reactive chemical compounds, including sugars, aldehydes, and activated oxygen species) are some of the variables that influence kin aging. Changes in skin structure, function, and appearance are the result of all these forces working together. However, there is little doubt that the main cause of skin aging is solar UV radiation.

Stimulation of Collagen and Elastin Production Many antiaging treatments work by stimulating the production of collagen and elastin in the skin. These proteins are essential for maintaining skin structure, elasticity, and firmness. Procedures such as microneedling, laser therapy, and certain topical treatments, such as retinoids and growth factors, can promote collagen and elastin synthesis, leading to smoother, more youthful-looking skin.

Exfoliation and Cell Turnover Exfoliation helps remove dead skin cells and encourages cell turnover, revealing younger-looking skin below. It is therefore an important step in the fight against skin aging. The skin is exfoliated with the aid of chemical peels, microdermabrasion, and exfoliating chemicals such as beta hydroxy acids (BHAs) and alpha hydroxy acids (AHAs), which decrease the visibility of age spots, wrinkles, and fine lines.

Protection Against UV Damage One of the main causes of early skin aging is UV radiation from the sun. Antioxidants (including vitamins C and E), DNA repair enzymes, and broad-spectrum sunscreens are examples of substances that shield the skin from UV ray damage and are frequently used in antiaging therapies. These components lessen inflammation, minimize the development of wrinkles and hyperpigmentation caused by UV exposure, and stop collagen deterioration.

Optimal Skin Moisture Preserving skin health and reducing signs of aging require maintaining a sufficient level of skin moisture. Antiaging skincare products often contain hyaluronic acid, glycerin, and other humectants to draw and hold moisture in the skin, improving its supply, plumpness, and texture.

Anti-Inflammatory Effects Accelerated skin aging is linked to chronic inflammation. To calm irritated skin, reduce redness, and stop collagen degradation, antiaging therapies may include anti-inflammatory substances such as niacinamide, green tea extract, and liquorice root extract.

In general, a number of strategies work together to reduce the appearance of aging skin indicators. These strategies include increasing the synthesis of collagen and elastin, encouraging exfoliation and cell turnover, guarding against UV ray damage, improving skin hydration, lowering inflammation, and blocking MMP activity. To produce antiaging benefits, many therapies may focus on one or more of these processes.

2.4 Histological and Immunohistochemical Evaluation

We may evaluate the effectiveness of mesotherapy on histological alterations, such as variations in the concentration of freshly synthesized collagen, via histological examination.

On the other hand, quantitative assessments using immunochemistry and histochemistry of collagen types I, III, and VII, freshly synthesized collagen, total elastin, and tropoelastin were carried out to gauge the effectiveness of numerous fractional erbium laser sessions for skin rejuvenation.

In a clinical study published in 2016, the purpose of this study was to assess the safety and effectiveness of intradermal platelet-rich plasma (PRP) injections for facial rejuvenation in humans.

Over the past few years, platelet-rich plasma (PRP) has been employed as an efficient therapy in a number of surgical and medical specialties. Publications regarding the application of PRP in orthopedic and trauma surgery, burn therapy, maxillofacial surgery, soft tissue injuries, periodontal and oral surgery, wound care, and gastrointestinal procedures are available. They reported an increase in the number and thickness of elastic fibers in the PRP and saline sites.

Collagen fiber bundles in the dermis were more numerous at the PRP and saline sites than at the pretreatment site. Increases in the quantity and thickness of elastic fibers in PRP and saline.

Vascular endothelial growth factor (VEGF), transforming growth factor (TGF), plaque-derived growth factor (PDGF), and insulin-like growth factor (IGF) are among the growth factors released from aggregation inducers (18) that stimulate concentrated platelet α-granules. These α-granules contain approximately 30 bioactive chemicals. Numerous surface receptors are expressed by fibroblasts, which are also capable of concurrently sensing several chemicals that cause behavioral reactions.

Following injection into the target tissue, a variety of growth factors and cytokines that promote the buildup of the extracellular matrix (ECM) and enhance cell proliferation and differentiation are triggered. Angiogenesis, migration, and proliferation of cells lead to tissue regeneration.

Through the breakdown of collagen and extracellular matrix proteins, matrix metalloproteinase (MMP) proteins contribute to the aging process.

Kim et al.'s research focused on the remodeling of the extracellular matrix (ECM), a process that necessitates dermal fibroblast activation.

They discovered that in human dermal fibroblasts, PRP increased the expression of type I collagen, MMP-1, and mRNA. PRP stimulates fibroblasts to produce new collagen.

According to Kakudo et al.'s research, the addition of activated platelet-rich or platelet-poor plasma considerably accelerated the growth of human dermal fibroblasts and adipose-derived stem cells in cell culture.

Cho et al. assessed the impact of the PRP. They propose that PRP causes human skin fibroblasts to express more type I collagen, MMP-1, and MMP-2. In another study, Kakudo et al.examined the duration until epithelialization and discomfort during gauze change by conducting a half-sided test comparing the PRP-treated and control (untreated) sides of a split-thickness skin transplant donor site. They discovered that in donor locations for split-thickness skin grafts, PRP stimulates angiogenesis and epithelialization. According to these in vitro experimental investigations, PRP promotes wound healing through fibroblast proliferation, collagen production, angiogenesis, and epithelialization.

Snehal P et al. reported that, from a mean of 59 to 48 nm, the mean diameter of the collagen fibers decreased. Smaller collagen molecules are commonly linked to type III collagen or procollagens, as well as the manufacture of new collagen. Freshly synthesized collagen responds to a variety of stimuli, such as heat or inflammatory damage, and is commonly linked to the existence of a healing zone.

It is quite probable that the most fundamental type of mesotherapy has no appreciable effect on the ultrastructural, histologic, or clinical characteristics of collagen fibers. They reported that there were no notable histopathological or long-term clinical consequences noted. Given that the total treatment value determined by temporal sequencing photographs in pairs is only a way to assess any advantage (or damage), the absolute value does not reflect the size of the effect.

2.5 Clinical Applications

As our chapter is about mesotherapy and skin reinventor, it is worth noting that mesotherapy has been used for other purposes.

Cellulite reduction: Injections are sometimes used to target cellulite, helping to break down fat deposits and improve the appearance of dimpled skin.

Hair Loss: Mesotherapy injections may be used to stimulate hair growth and improve the health of the scalp.

Body Contouring: This method is sometimes employed to target specific areas of the body where localized fat deposits are present through lipolytic mesotherapy.

The basis of lipolytic immunotherapy is the induction of lipolysis in adipocytes. Initially, mesotherapy for lipolytic stimulation was predicated on empirical findings. In vitro tests utilizing various lipolytic stimulators that misanthropists frequently use have been carried out more recently. On the basis of body location, in vivo research, including lipolytic mesotherapy, can be further split. Women have long complained that it is harder to immobilize fat on the hips and thighs, but the scientific community did not accept these empirical data. These findings have since been verified by scholars, and it is known that the relative lipolytic thresholds of fat cells in various body regions dictate an individual's distribution of fat.

One recent randomized clinical trial (RCT) mentioned the role of mesotherapy in the management of spinal pain. Mesotherapy may be viewed as a helpful auxiliary in pain treatment facilities as well as a tailored strategy in general practitioner settings.

In 2015, Aurora Tedeschi et al. validated the potential benefit of HA mesotherapy for the treatment of photoaging and skin aging, as demonstrated by quantified ultrasound data demonstrating notable temporal changes in subepidermal low-echogenic band (SLEB) density.

2.5.1 Reliving Pain

As we mentioned previously, mesh therapy can be administered through injections either (intradermal or subcutaneous) and can lead to some pain in the patient; some common ways to relieve pain are as follow

1. **Cold Compress:** Ice or a cold compress should be applied to reduce inflammation and reduce pain.
2. **Over-the-**counter pain medications: Nonprescription pain relievers such as acetaminophen or ibuprofen following recommended dosages should be used.
3. **Topical Anesthetics:** N numbing creams or gels with lidocaine or benzocaine were applied to the treated area.
4. **Arnica Montana:** Use arnica gel or cream with anti-inflammatory properties to reduce pain and swelling.
5. **Follow Post-Care Instructions:** Adhere to guidelines provided by your healthcare provider for optimal healing and pain management.

Firas Al-Qarqaz et al. mentioned another way to reduce pain; 40 patients who received skin injections were included. For the same patient, the visual analog scale (VAS) was used to assess the patient's pain level both with and without cold air. A comparison of the pain ratings was performed. When cold air was used, 33 patients' VAS scores decreased. Two patients experienced no change in their pain level, and five individuals had worse VAS ratings overall. There was a considerably greater decrease in the patient group (n = 5) receiving injections to the palms. in VAS ratings. No notable negative effects occurred either immediately or later.

2.6 Clinical Assessment Tools for Facial Rejuvenation

2.6.1 *Face Visual Scale*

The subjective facial visual scale is a tool used to gauge patient happiness. On a 0–10 scale, six particular studies have demonstrated a statistically significant mean improvement in individuals undergoing skin treatments such as hyaluronic acid.

2.6.2 *Wrinkle Severity Rating Scale WSRS*

The scale has been verified and has a maximum wrinkle severity of 1 and a maximum wrinkle severity of 5. The highest degree of intensity, where 1 denotes absence, 2 mild, 3 moderate, 4 severe, and 5 extremes.

The WSRS was utilized by blinded investigators, and Calabaro et al. examined it and reported that it is a reliable quantitative evaluation with strong intra- and interobserver agreement. Furthermore, two dermatologists compared GAIS before and after surgery in a study published by Lee et al.

The effectiveness of treating NLFs via hydroxypropyl methylcellulose (HPMC) and polymethylmethacrylate cross-linked dextran (PMMA) was evaluated.

To evaluate the safety and effectiveness of L-polylactic acid in the treatment of facial aging, one study exclusively employed photos.

To measure improvements in various skin changes, including wrinkles, hyperpigmentation, pore size, and other cosmetic aspects, the authors have coupled invasive or noninvasive procedures with a variety of quantitative methodologies for objective assessments. Among the several objective techniques applied, we observed this phenomenon.

2.7 New Advancements in Mesotherapy

Mesotherapy, when combined with technology and artificial intelligence (AI), is a revolutionary new development in medical aesthetics and customized skincare. With the introduction of innovative technology and AI algorithms, mesotherapy—a minimally invasive cosmetic surgery that involves injecting different chemicals into the mesoderm—has undergone a revolutionary change. Advanced imaging technologies allow mesotherapy practitioners to precisely target certain skin layers and optimize drug distribution, which is one way that technology plays a crucial role in improving precision and safety during treatment. Customized mesotherapy procedures may be created by AI algorithms using machine learning to evaluate enormous databases of patient data, skin types, and treatment results. With fewer possible negative effects, our customized strategy guarantees the best possible outcomes.

Furthermore, with the amalgamation of intelligent gadgets and surveillance systems, this customized strategy minimizes any negative effects while guaranteeing the best possible outcomes. Furthermore, real-time tracking of patient reactions and treatment plan modifications are made possible by the integration of smart devices and monitoring systems. The combination of AI and technology in mesotherapy simplifies procedures while simultaneously creating new opportunities for innovation. This heralds a new age in aesthetic medicine, where tailored treatments are informed by technological precision and data-driven insights.

Lingling Hu et al. reported that the clinical effect of mesotherapy with a nanochip device could involve the use of sensors for real-time monitoring, ensuring accurate placement of therapeutic substances and allowing for adjustments on the basis of individual skin responses. For facial rejuvenation, the brightness and texture of the skin can be improved with the use of mesotherapy nanochips, but the results are temporary. For patients in need of facial rejuvenation, it is advised that the procedure be utilized in addition to other methods.

2.8 Mesotherapy Instructions

See Tables 2.1 and 2.2.

2.9 Ethical Considerations

Ethics is a critical aspect that needs to be covered to safely include mesotherapy in each patient's personalized treatment plan and to accurately explain the method to health authorities' decision-makers.

Table 2.1 Pre-treatment

Time period	Action
10 days or longer before treatment	– Stay away from supplements containing willow bark or gingko biloba
5 days before starting therapy	– Avoid aspirin, vitamin E, and over-the-counter pain relievers (e.g., Aleve, Advil, or Motrin)
Day before treatment	– Cut back on coffee
Day of treatment	– Avoid taking any prescription stimulants
3 days before treatment (for facial)	– Begin taking your Medrol dosage pack
Morning before treatment	– Use antibacterial soap to wash the treated region thoroughly
Before treatment (except for face)	– Avoid using creams, lotions, sprays, or bath oils on the areas to be treated
At least 2 h before treatment	– Use Arnica cream (unless it is being applied to the face)

Table 2.2 Posttreatment instructions

Time period	Action
After treatment	– Steer clear of hot showers or baths for at least 48 h
Day of treatment	– Consume a gallon of water
After treatment (ongoing)	– Consume at least 80 ounces of water (10 glasses) every day until all treatments are completed
For at least 2 weeks posttreatment	– Avoid saunas and hot pools (above 102°)
48 h after treatment	– Allow a 48-h period without intense activity
Two to three days posttreatment	– Continue using Arnica cream three to four times a day
48 h after treatment	– Avoid applying any additional creams or lotions to the treated regions
At least 48 h posttreatment	– Wear loose-fitting clothing
Following treatment	– Keep in mind that bruises may persist for 10 days or longer following therapy

To accomplish these objectives, we must evaluate the available data via a methodology grounded in scientific integrity. M. Mammucari et al. -2021- In his study in an Italian population, it is essential to take the time required to explain to the patient the reasoning behind this decision, the reasons behind the selection of a particular medication (particularly if it is off-label), and the anticipated distinction in comparison to alternative administration methods. Additionally, we advise mentioning the type of therapy received and the outcomes in the medical records. Additionally, we affirm the necessity of ad hoc professional training on the basis of scientific data rather than subjective ideas passed down from one doctor to another with statements 28 and 29. Before this study, none of these were considered mesotherapy.

They advise against self-administration for cosmetic reasons, specifically because dermal infiltration can also have serious repercussions if it is not performed in a hygienic manner or in an appropriate setting. For all of these reasons, we highly advise adhering to hygiene guidelines (statements 8 and 9).

Further Reading

1. Bhawan J, Andersen W, Lee J, et al. Photo aging versus intrinsic aging: a morphologic assessment of facial skin. J Cutan Pathol. 1995;22:154–9.
2. Iorizzo M, De Padova MP, Tosti A. Biorejuvenation: theory and practice. Clin Dermatol. 2008;26(2):177–81.
3. Kandhari R, Kaur I, Sharma D. Mesococktails and mesoproducts in aesthetic dermatology. Dermatol Ther. 2020;33(6):e14218. https://doi.org/10.1111/dth.14218.
4. Sivagnanam G. Mesotherapy—The French Connection [Internet]. https://www.ncbi.nlm.nih.gov/pmc/articles/PMC3142757/.
5. Jayasinghe S, Guillot T, Bissoon L, Greenway F. Mesotherapy for local fat reduction. Obes Rev. 2013;14(10):780–91.

6. Fanian F, Deutsch JJ, Bousquet MT, Boisnic S, Andre P, Catoni I, et al. A hyaluronic acid-based microfiller improves superficial wrinkles and skin quality: a randomized prospective controlled multicenter study. J Dermatol Treat. 2023;34(1):2216323.
7. Bazargan AS, Shemshadi M, Ziaeifar E, Taheri A, Roohaninasab M, Goodarzi A, et al. Evaluation of effectiveness of tranexamic acid as mesotherapy in improvement of periorbital wrinkling in a trial study. J Cosmet Dermatol. 2023;22(9):2548–52.
8. Zasada M, Markiewicz A, Drożdż Z, Mosińska P, Erkiert-Polguj A, Budzisz E. Preliminary randomized controlled trial of antiaging effects of l-ascorbic acid applied in combination with no-needle and microneedle mesotherapy. J Cosmet Dermatol. 2019;18(3):843–9.
9. Rittié L, Fisher GJ. UV-light-induced signal cascades and skin aging. Ageing Res Rev. 1:704.
10. Fisher GJ, Kang S, Varani J, Bata-Csorgo Z, Wan Y, Datta S, Voorhees JJ. Mechanisms of photoaging and chronological skin aging. Arch Dermatol. 2002;138:1462.
11. Mukherjee S, Date A, Patravale V, Korting HC, Roeder A, Weindl G. Retinoids in the treatment of skin aging: an overview of clinical efficacy and safety. Clin Interv Aging. 2006;1(4):327–48.
12. Baumann L. Skin aging and its treatment. J Pathol. 2007;211:241.
13. Leyden JJ, Shergill B, Micali G, Downie J, Wallo W. Natural options for the management of hyperpigmentation. J Eur Acad Dermatol Venereol. 2011;25:1140.
14. Levin J, Rosso JQD, Momin SB. How much do we truly know about our favorite cosmeceutical ingredients? J Clin Aesthet Dermatol. 2010;3(2):22.
15. El-Domyati M, El-Ammawi TS, Medhat W, Moawad O, Mahoney MG, Uitto J. Multiple minimally invasive erbium: yttrium aluminum garnet laser mini-peels for skin rejuvenation: an objective assessment. J Cosmet Dermatol. 2012;11(2):122–30.
16. Redaelli A, Romano D, Marcianó A. Face and neck revitalization with platelet-rich plasma (PRP): clinical outcome in a series of 23 consecutively treated patients. J Drugs Dermatol. 2010;9:466.
17. Abuaf OK, Yildiz H, Baloglu H, Bilgili ME, Simsek HA, Dogan B. Histologic evidence of new collagen formulation using platelet rich plasma in skin rejuvenation: a prospective controlled clinical study. Ann Dermatol. 2016;28(6):718–24.
18. Kim DH, Je YJ, Kim CD, Lee YH, Seo YJ, Lee JH, et al. Can platelet-rich plasma be used for skin rejuvenation? Evaluation of effects of platelet-rich plasma on human dermal fibroblast. Ann Dermatol. 2011;23(4):424–31.
19. Çayırlı M, Çalışkan E, Açıkgöz G, Erbil AH, Ertürk G. Regression of melasma with platelet-rich plasma treatment. Ann Dermatol. 2014;26(3):401–2.
20. Anitua E, Sánchez M, Zalduendo MM, De La Fuente M, Prado R, Orive G, et al. Fibroblastic response to treatment with different preparations rich in growth factors. Cell Prolif. 2009;42(2):162–70.
21. Banihashemi M, Nakhaeizadeh S. An introduction to application of platelet rich plasma (PRP) in skin rejuvenation. Rev Clin Med. 2014;1:38.
22. Kakudo N, Kushida S, Minakata T, Suzuki K, Kusumoto K. Platelet-rich plasma promotes epithelialization and angiogenesis in a splitthickness skin graft donor site. Med Mol Morphol. 2011;44:233.
23. Cho J-W, Kim S-A, Lee K-S. Platelet-rich plasma induces increased expression of G1 cell cycle regulators, type I collagen, and matrix metalloproteinase-1 in human skin fibroblasts. Int J Mol Med. 2012;29:32.
24. Amin SP, Phelps RG, Goldberg DJ. Mesotherapy for facial skin rejuvenation: a clinical, histologic, and electron microscopic evaluation. Dermatol Surg. 2006;32(12):1467–72.
25. Schmults CD, Phelps R, Goldberg DJ. Nonablative facial remodeling: erythema reduction and histologic evidence of new collagen formation using a 300-microsecond 1064-nm Nd:YAG laser. Arch Dermatol. 2004;140(11):1373. https://doi.org/10.1001/archderm.140.11.1373.
26. Laurent A, Mistretta F, Bottigioli D, Dahel K, Goujon C, Nicolas JF, et al. Echographic measurement of skin thickness in adults by high frequency ultrasound to assess the appropriate microneedle length for intradermal delivery of vaccines. Vaccine. 2007;25(34):6423–30.

27. Kakasheva-Mazhenkovska L. Variations of the histomorphological characteristics of human skin of different body regions in subjects of different age. https://pubmed.ncbi.nlm.nih.gov/22286617/.
28. Thappa D, Konda D. Mesotherapy: what is new? Indian J Dermatol Venereol Leprol. 2013;79(1):127.
29. Lacarrubba F, Tedeschi A, Nardone B, Micali G. Mesotherapy for skin rejuvenation: assessment of the subepidermal low-echogenic band by ultrasound evaluation with cross-sectional B-mode scanning. Dermatol Ther. 2008;21:S1–5.
30. Smith U, Hammersten J, Björntorp P, Kral JG. Regional differences and effect of weight reduction on human fat cell metabolism. Eur J Clin Invest. 1979;9(5):327–32.
31. Brauneis S, Araimo F, Rossi M. The role of mesotherapy in the management of spinal pain. A randomized controlled study. Clin Ter. 2023;4:336–42.
32. Tedeschi A, Lacarrubba F, Micali G. Mesotherapy with an intradermal hyaluronic acid formulation for skin rejuvenation: an intrapatient, placebo-controlled, long-term trial using high-frequency ultrasound. Aesthet Plast Surg. 2015;39(1):129–33.
33. Buntrock H, Reuther T, Prager W, Kerscher M. Efficacy, safety, and patient satisfaction of a monophasic cohesive polydensified matrix versus a biphasic nonanimal stabilized hyaluronic acid filler after single injection in nasolabial folds. Dermatol Surg. 2013;39:1097.
34. Calabrò G, De Vita V, Patalano A, Mazzella C, Conte VL, Antropoli C. Confirmed efficacy of topical nifedipine in the treatment of facial wrinkles. J Dermatol Treat. 2014;25:319.
35. Lee YB, Song EJ, Kim SS, Kim JW, Yu DS. Safety and efficacy of a novel injectable filler in the treatment of nasolabial folds: polymethylmethacrylate and cross-linked dextran in hydroxypropyl methylcellulose. J Cosmet Laser Ther. 2014;16:185.
36. Olivier Masveyraud F. Facial rejuvenation using L-polylactic acid: approximately 298 successive cases. Ann Chir Plast Esthet. 2011;56:120.
37. Hu L, Zhao K, Song WM. Effect of mesotherapy with nanochip in the treatment of facial rejuvenation. J Cosmet Laser Ther. 2020;22(2):84–9.
38. FDA allows marketing of first whole slide imaging system for digital pathology. https://www.fda.gov/news-events/press-announcements/fda-allows-marketing-first-whole-slide-imaging-system-digital-pathology.
39. Wells A, Patel S, Lee JB, Motaparthi K. Artificial intelligence in dermatopathology: diagnosis, education, and research. J Cutan Pathol. 2021;48(8):1061–8.
40. Babacan T, Onat AM, Pehlivan Y, Comez G, Tutar E. A case of the Behcet's disease diagnosed by the panniculits after mesotherapy. Rheumatol Int. 2010;30(12):1657–9.
41. Galmés-Truyols A, Giménez-Duran J, Bosch-Isabel C, Nicolau-Riutort A, Vanrell-Berga J, Portell-Arbona M, et al. An outbreak of cutaneous infection due to mycobacterium abscessus associated with mesotherapy. Enfermedades Infecc Microbiol Clínica. 2011;29(7):510–4.
42. Correa NE, Cataño JC, Mejía GI, Realpe T, Orozco B, Estrada S, Vélez A, Vélez L, Barón P, Guzmán A, Robledo J. Outbreak of mesotherapy-associated cutaneous infections caused by Mycobacterium chelonae in Colombia. Jpn J Infect Dis. 2010;63:143.
43. Alejandra Rivera-Olivero I, Guevara A, Escalona A, Oliver M, Pérez-Alfonzo R, Piquero J, et al. Infecciones en tejidos blandos por micobacterias no tuberculosas secundarias a mesoterapia. ¿Cuánto vale la belleza? Enfermedades Infecc Microbiol Clínica. 2006;24(5):302–6.
44. Mammucari M, Russo D, Maggiori E. Evidence-based recommendations on mesotherapy: an update from the Italian Society of Mesotherapy. Clin Ter. 2021;171:37–45.
45. Mesotherapy pre and post treatment instructions. https://cosmetiqmedicine.com/wp-content/uploads/kybella-fat-dissolving-pre_post-instructions.pdf.

Chapter 3
Role of Mesotherapy in Dermatological Disorders

Therese Anne Limbana, Caleb Sooknanan and Esraa M. AlEdani

3.1 Introduction

Mesotherapy is a term that is derived from the Greek words "mesos" (middle) and "therapeia" (to treat medically). This treatment was first described by Michel Pistor in Europe. Currently, it is gaining popularity for the treatment of various skin disorders and the rejuvenation of skin. Although most of the ingredients used in mesotherapy are approved by the U.S. Food and Drug Administration (FDA), some are currently being used because they are not yet approved. Mesotherapy is a noninvasive approach that involves the transdermal injection of vitamins, hormones, plant extracts, enzymes, and hyaluronic acid. Different injection techniques are used in mesotherapy, including the intraepidermal technique, injection into the dermoepidermal junction, injection at a depth of 2–4 mm (nappage), and injection into the deep dermis. The most common applications of mesotherapy are skin rejuvenation, acne treatment, and melasma.

Mesotherapy uses sterile water-soluble substances, including minerals, antioxidants, and vitamins, which are suitable for intradermal injection. Furthermore, each substance must be injected separately in different syringes to ensure efficacy and safety. Mesotherapy involves penetrating the epidermal barrier either through direct injection or microporous introduction to deliver cosmetically active ingredients directly into the dermis or deeper subcutaneous layers. In this way, mesotherapy accelerates skin metabolism, thus improving skin quality from the inside out. The main principle of mesotherapy is based on a simple skin healing process following trauma.

T. A. Limbana · C. Sooknanan
New York Institute of Technology College of Osteopathic Medicine, Glen Head, NY, USA

E. M. AlEdani (✉)
Basra Medical College, Basrah, Iraq

E. M. AlEdani, H. Maibach (eds.), *Mesotherapy and Its Medical Applications*, Updates in Clinical Dermatology, https://doi.org/10.1007/978-3-031-76070-9_3

For dermatological disorders, mesotherapy uses this method of trauma and repair. Furthermore, mesotherapy enhances drug absorption rates by effectively breaking down the epidermis, thereby allowing drug treatments to attain greater efficacy. Currently, a limited number of studies have been published on the use of mesotherapy for the treatment of various dermatological disorders. Furthermore, the efficacy described in these studies also varies. This chapter looks for scientific evidence that shows the effectiveness of mesotherapy in the treatment of various dermatological conditions.

3.2 Mesotherapy for Acne

Acne vulgaris is a common cutaneous inflammatory disease that affects mostly adults; however, it can also be reported in children and teenagers. Patients with acne are quite prone to experiencing the recurrence of acne attacks, which are associated with adverse consequences for mental health. The use of mesotherapy for acne treatment has been relatively less studied. Some studies have reported that mesotherapy has better efficacy than standard treatment modalities for acne. In their study, Chen et al. investigated the effectiveness of mesotherapy with the compound glycyrrhizin in the treatment of acne. They compared mesotherapy with clindamycin gel. The study included 108 patients, who were equally divided into treatment and control groups. Their findings revealed that, compared with conventional treatment with clindamycin gel, mesotherapy treatment for acne had superior results. Furthermore, mesotherapy was associated with reduced loss of skin moisture and better integrity of the skin barrier. Mesotherapy also inhibited inflammatory reactions in patients. Postinflammatory erythema (PAE) is a sequela of acne that can disturb patients even after the resolution of acne. Mesotherapy has been shown to improve PAE symptoms in patients. Bazargan et al. used tranexamic acid (TA) as a mesotherapy for the treatment of PAE. The treatment involved two sessions of mesotherapy at 2-week intervals. The treatment was applied to the right side, whereas the left side was used as a control. Following treatment, the difference was recorded with photographs. The findings revealed that after mesotherapy treatment, there was a significant difference in the number, percentage, and area of PAE lesions. However, no change was observed in the left-side control area.

Mesotherapy can also be used in combination with other treatment modalities. The use of mesotherapy in combination with 20% glycol acid has been reported. A 33-year-old female with acne scars was treated with four sessions of mesotherapy in combination with glycol acid. Following treatment, the patient experienced reduced inflammation and a decreased number of acne scars. Another case study used mesenchymal stem cell-containing placenta extract solution for mesotherapy in patients with acne. Their findings revealed that following treatment, there was an 80% improvement in acne scars and complexion of the skin. There was also improvement in the number of icepicks and rolling scars. Mesenchymal stem cells (MSCs) have great therapeutic effects on tissue regeneration. The primary mechanism through which MSCs contribute to tissue regeneration lies in their ability to secrete a wide range of bioactive trophic factors. These factors play crucial roles in stimulating adjacent parenchymal cells to initiate the repair of damaged tissues. They influence the local immune response, promote the formation of new blood vessels, inhibit cell apoptosis, and promote the survival, proliferation, and differentiation of resident tissue-specific cells.

3.3 Mesotherapy for Melasma

Melasma is a pigmentary disorder that commonly occurs on the face. The hyperpigmented patches have irregular borders and are mostly restricted to sun-exposed areas. One of the primary difficulties in treating melasma is the inadequate absorption and impermeability of water-soluble substances through the thick and hydrophobic stratum corneum. This barrier results in a poor response of dermal or mixed types of melasma to topical treatments. The pathogenesis of melasma is not understood; however, increased melanin production and melanocytes are involved in hyperpigmentation in melasma. Ultraviolet (UV) radiation is the most aggravating factor that triggers melanocytosis and melanogenesis. This process occurs through the induction of plasminogen activator synthesis and the subsequent increase in plasmin activity within keratinocytes. Tranexamic acid (TA) has been used in many studies because it is a plasmin inhibitor. It is a lysine analog that functions by temporarily inhibiting lysine binding sites on plasminogen molecules. This action leads to a reduction in melanocyte activity. Consequently, TA has gained popularity in recent treatments for melasma because of its ability to diminish hyperpigmentation. However, the efficacy of topical and oral TA is not high and is associated with systemic side effects, particularly if TA is taken for longer durations. A pilot study used TA mesotherapy for melasma treatment, with a dose ranging from 150–200 mg/session for TA. Following treatment, the melanin index gradually improved by the 8th week, with a statistically significant decrease observed by the 16th week. For the modified Melasma Area and Severity Index (mMASI) score, a reduction was noted by the 4th week, with statistically significant decreases recorded at the 8th, 12th, and 16th weeks. Specifically, the mMASI score decreased by 0.99 (36.26%) at week 8, 1.56 (57.14%) at week 12, and 1.50 (54.95%) at week 16. By the 16th week, both the mMASI score and the melanin index significantly decreased compared with those at baseline. Furthermore, there were no systemic side effects of the treatment. The effectiveness of TA mesotherapy has also been compared with that of hydroquinone (HQ) cream. The patients in the mesotherapy groups were treated with 4 mg/mL or 10 mg/mL TA. Posttreatment, there was a significant reduction in the MASI score at the 12th week compared with baseline. When the results were compared with those of the 4% HQ cream, there was a significant reduction in the MASI score compared with that of the 4 mg/mL mesotherapy treatment. Similarly, the use of mesotherapy in combination with HQ 4% cream has also been shown to provide greater benefits than does the use of HQ 4% cream alone (20.96% vs. 14.11%).

In an open-label randomized controlled trial (RCT), the effectiveness of oral TA (250 mg twice daily for 12 weeks) was compared with that of TA mesotherapy (4 mg/cc, administered over 3 monthly sessions). The results revealed a notable disparity in efficacy, with oral TXA yielding a significantly greater rate of good-to-excellent improvement than ID injection did (99.99% versus 52.75%, respectively). However, in a comparative analysis conducted by Shetty et al., a substantially greater reduction in the mMASI score was observed with TA microinjection (4 mg/cc) than with oral administration (35.6% versus 21.7%, respectively). Furthermore, enhanced efficacy was particularly prominent among female patients, younger patients, and individuals with lighter skin phototypes. Patil et al. reported that with TA mesotherapy, there was a 71.6% improvement in the MASI score compared with 33.3% with oral TA. Similarly, another RCT revealed that compared with 10% TA cream (4.2%), mesotherapy with 4 mg/cc and 10 mg/cc resulted in significant improvements (39.1% and 62.7%, respectively). With increasing doses of TA, some studies have reported better benefits. For example, when the dose of TA mesotherapy was increased to 20 mg/cc, the treatment was more effective than HQ 2% cream was. Similarly, a higher concentration (100 mg/cc) of TA mesotherapy showed much better efficacy than HQ (4%). Similarly, mesotherapy can also be used in combination with ablative lasers. A study by Tawfic et al. compared the effectiveness of combining a fractional carbon dioxide laser (FCO2) with TA mesotherapy at a concentration of 100 mg/cc with that of using FCO2 in combination with topical TA or FCO2 alone. The findings of the study revealed that the combination of laser and ID injection resulted in a greater improvement in the melanin index (MI) than did laser therapy alone. Another study reported that compared with Er:YAG laser therapy, mesotherapy with TA significantly reduced the MASI score. Greater than 75% improvement was recorded in the group that received mesotherapy (29.6%) compared with the Er:YAG laser group (11.1%).

In addition to TA, vitamin C, glutathione, and triamcinolone are also commonly used for the treatment of melasma. Some studies have demonstrated the efficacy of different combinations of mesotherapies as well. For example, one study used a combination of TA with 3% vitamin C and 2% glutathione and compared it with TA and a 3% vitamin C combination. However, they reported that triple combination therapy resulted in more edema and ecchymosis than did double combination therapy. Triamcinolone has beneficial effects on melasma, as it reduces melanogenesis by inhibiting inflammatory mediators. Previous studies have shown that triamcinolone (4 mg/cc) significantly reduces the MASI score after mesotherapy treatment compared with baseline. Vitamin C, also known as ascorbic acid, and glutathione are both antioxidants with anti-inflammatory properties. They work by blocking the tyrosinase enzyme, which is involved in melanin production, and by reducing harmful reactive oxygen species (ROS). Additionally, vitamin C helps strengthen the skin barrier and promotes the production of collagen. Studies have shown promising results with these treatments. Puri et al. reported that a combination of vitamin C and glutathione injections led to a significant improvement in skin pigmentation, with more than 75% of patients experiencing a greater than half reduction in pigmentation scores after 6 months of treatment. Similarly, in a randomized controlled trial, Balevi et al. reported a greater reduction in pigmentation scores when vitamin C mesotherapy was added to salicylic acid peel treatments than when the peel alone was used. However, the difference between the two groups was not significant after 6 months.

3.4 Mesotherapy for Rosacea

Rosacea is a chronic condition that is characterized by facial redness, visible blood vessels, and occasional, pus-filled bumps on the skin. It primarily affects central facial features and may be associated with burning or stinging sensations, dry skin and potential swelling. While its exact cause is still under investigation, rosacea presents with more severe symptoms on a periodic basis. Recent studies suggest that mesotherapy may be used to address rosacea symptoms. For example, Bharti et al. suggested that mesotherapy consisting of topical and systemic antibiotics, azelaic acid, tranexamic acid, isoretinoin, chemical peels, and intensely pulsed light therapy may improve the papulopustular components of rosacea, which would decrease the appearance of lesions on patients' scalps and faces. However, vascular symptoms associated with edema, flushing, and persistent erythema persisted. More work is needed to understand how mesotherapy can address other aspects of the presentation of rosacea.

3.5 Mesotherapy for Androgenetic Alopecia

Androgenetic alopecia is the most frequent cause of hair loss and is often associated with decreases in scalp hair density due to hair follicle miniaturization. Saceda-Corralo et al. suggested that mesotherapy with dutasteride could be used to improve hair loss and reduce systemic absorption associated with alopecia. The side effects related to the treatment were mild, so further work would allow clinicians to develop more effective mesotherapy options for alopecia.

3.6 Conclusion

In conclusion, mesotherapy has good efficacy in the treatment of various dermatological conditions. The utilization of mesotherapy is particularly beneficial in conditions that are difficult to treat with standard modalities. Furthermore, mesotherapy can be used in combination with other treatments to further increase the benefits.

Further Reading

1. De Padova MP, Fabbrocini G, Cacciapuoti S, Tosti A. Mesotherapy. Textbook of cosmetic dermatology. Boca Raton, FL: CRC; 2017. p. 443–7.
2. Al Faresi F, Galadari HI. Mesotherapy: myth and reality. Expert Rev Dermatol. 2011;6(2):157–62.
3. El-Domyati M, El-Ammawi TS, Moawad O, El-Fakahany H, Medhat W, Mahoney MG, et al. Efficacy of mesotherapy in facial rejuvenation: a histological and immunohistochemical evaluation. Int J Dermatol. 2012;51(8):913–9.
4. Plachouri KM, Georgiou S. Mesotherapy: safety profile and management of complications. J Cosmet Dermatol. 2019;18(6):1601–5.
5. Mammucari M, Maggiori E, Russo D, Giorgio C, Ronconi G, Ferrara PE, et al. Mesotherapy: from historical notes to scientific evidence and future prospects. ScientificWorldJournal. 2020;2020:3542848–9.
6. Khalili M, Amiri R, Iranmanesh B, Zartab H, Aflatoonian M. Safety and efficacy of mesotherapy in the treatment of melasma: a review article. J Cosmet Dermatol. 2022;21(1):118–29.
7. Natsuaki MN, Yates TM. Adolescent acne and disparities in mental health. Child Dev Perspect. 2021;15(1):37–43.
8. Chen Y, Han W, Li S, Nie Y, Chen P, Sun J, et al. Effects of mesotherapy introduction of compound glycyrrhizin injection on the treatment of moderate to severe acne. J Cosmet Dermatol. 2023;22(7):1973–9.
9. Bazargan AS, Ziaeifar E, Abouie A, Mirahmadi S, Taheri A, Gheisari M. Evaluating the effect of tranexamic acid as mesotherapy on persistent postacne erythema: a before and after study. J Cosmet Dermatol. 2023;22(10):2714–20.
10. Chilicka K, Pagacz K. The use of combination therapy with 20% glycolic acid and fractional mesotherapy to reduce acne scars: a case report. Med Sci Pulse. 2019;13(2):49–51.
11. Phonchai R, Naigowit P, Ubonsaen B, Nilubol S, Brameld S, Noisa P. Improvement of atrophic acne scar and skin complexity by combination of aqueous human placenta extract and mesenchymal stem cell mesotherapy. J Cosmet Dermatol Sci Appl. 2020;10(1):1–7.
12. Najar M, Bouhtit F, Melki R, Afif H, Hamal A, Fahmi H, et al. Mesenchymal stromal cell-based therapy: new perspectives and challenges. J Clin Med. 2019;8(5):626.
13. Kamolz L-P, Keck M, Kasper C. Wharton's jelly mesenchymal stem cells promote wound healing and tissue regeneration. Stem Cell Res Ther. 2014;5:1–2.
14. Ogbechie-Godec OA, Elbuluk N. Melasma: an up-to-date comprehensive review. Dermatol Ther. 2017;7(3):305–18.
15. Shankar K, Godse K, Aurangabadkar S, Lahiri K, Mysore V, Ganjoo A, et al. Evidence-based treatment for melasma: expert opinion and a review. Dermatol Ther. 2014;4(2):165–86.
16. Hossain MR, Ansary TM, Komine M, Ohtsuki M. Diversified stimuli-induced inflammatory pathways cause skin pigmentation. Int J Mol Sci. 2021;22(8):3970.
17. Tse TW, Hui E. Tranexamic acid: an important adjuvant in the treatment of melasma. J Cosmet Dermatol. 2013;12(1):57–66.
18. Rodrigues M, Pandya AG. Melasma: clinical diagnosis and management options. Australas J Dermatol. 2015;56(3):151–63.
19. Wongwicharm P, Sirithanabadeekul P. The effectiveness of localized intradermal microinjection of 50 mg/ml of tranexamic acid for melasma treatment in Thai patients: a pilot study. Thai J Pharm Sci. 2018;42:93–7.
20. Pazyar N, Yaghoobi R, Zeynalie M, Vala S. Comparison of the efficacy of intradermal injected tranexamic acid vs hydroquinone cream in the treatment of melasma. Clin Cosmet Investig Dermatol. 2019;12:115–22.
21. Al-Hamamy HR, Aziz RM. The efficacy of intralesional tranexamic acid in the treatment of melasma in Iraqi patients. Iraq Postgrad Med J. 2020;19(2):127–32.

22. Khurana VK, Misri RR, Agarwal S, Thole AV, Kumar S, Anand T. A randomized, open-label, comparative study of oral tranexamic acid and tranexamic acid microinjections in patients with melasma. Indian J Dermatol Venereol Leprol. 2019;85(1):39–43.
23. Shetty VH, Shetty M. Comparative study of localized intradermal microinjection of tranexamic acid and oral tranexamic acid for the treatment of melasma. Int J Res Dermatol. 2018;4(3):363–7.
24. Patil S, Jamale V, Kale M, Nikam B, Hussain A, Vijayendran N. Safety and efficacy profile of oral tranexamic acid v/s tranexamic acid soaks v/s tranexamic acid cream in treatment of melasma—a hospital based prospective randomized controlled comparative study. JMSCR. 2018;6:151–62.
25. Badran AY, Ali AU, Gomaa AS. Efficacy of topical versus intradermal injection of tranexamic acid in Egyptian melasma patients: a randomized clinical trial. Australas J Dermatol. 2021;62(3):e373–e9.
26. Saki N, Darayesh M, Heiran A. Comparing the efficacy of topical hydroquinone 2% versus intradermal tranexamic acid microinjections in treating melasma: a split-face controlled trial. J Dermatol Treat. 2018;29(4):405–10.
27. Tehranchinia Z, Saghi B, Rahimi H. Evaluation of therapeutic efficacy and safety of tranexamic acid local infiltration in combination with topical 4% hydroquinone cream compared to topical 4% hydroquinone cream alone in patients with melasma: a split-face study. Dermatol Res Pract. 2018;2018:1–5.
28. Tawfic SO, Abdel Halim DM, Albarbary A, Abdelhady M. Assessment of combined fractional CO(2) and tranexamic acid in melasma treatment. Lasers Surg Med. 2019;51(1):27–33.
29. Otb S, Shaarawy E, Sadek A, Abdallah N, Agamia N, Soliman M, et al. A split face comparative study between intradermal tranexamic acid and erbium-YAG laser in treatment of melasma. J Dermatol Treat. 2022;33(1):555–9.
30. Iraji F, Nasimi M, Asilian A, Faghihi G, Mozafarpoor S, Hafezi H. Efficacy of mesotherapy with tranexamic acid and ascorbic acid with and without glutathione in treatment of melasma: a split face comparative trial. J Cosmet Dermatol. 2019;18(5):1416–21.
31. Eshghi G, Ashari FE. Comparison between intralesional triamcinolone and Kligman's formula in treatment of melasma. Acta Med Iran. 2016;54:67–71.
32. Nassar AAE, Ibrahim AM, Mahmoud AA. Efficacy and safety of intralesional steroid injection in the treatment of melasma. J Cosmet Dermatol. 2021;20(3):862–7.
33. Puri N. A study on the efficacy of mesotherapy using glutathione and vitamin C for the treatment of melasma. J Clin Exp Cosmet Dermatol. 2020;3(1):e005.
34. Balevi A, Ustuner P, Özdemir M. Salicylic acid peeling combined with vitamin C mesotherapy versus salicylic acid peeling alone in the treatment of mixed type melasma: a comparative study. J Cosmet Laser Ther. 2017;19(5):294–9.
35. Bharti J, Sonthalia S, Jakhar D. Mesotherapy with botulinum toxin for the treatment of refractory vascular and papulopustular rosacea. J Am Acad Dermatol. 2023;88(6):295–6.
36. Saceda-Corralo D, Moustafa F, Moreno-Arrones O, Jaén-Olasolo P, Vañó-Galván S, Camacho F. Mesotherapy with Dutasteride for androgenetic alopecia: a retrospective study in real clinical practice. J Drugs Dermatol. 2022;21(7):742–7.

Chapter 4
Role of Mesotherapy in Nondermatological Diseases

Esraa M. AlEdani

4.1 Mesotherapy and Pain

4.1.1 Mesotherapy

Mesotherapy involves the application of liquid mixtures (plant extracts, vitamins, and other components, as well as pharmaceutical and homoeopathic treatments) via intra- or subcutaneous injections for the treatment of specific local medical and cosmetic disorders. As an additional treatment for the management of localized pain, mesotherapy, also known as intradermal therapy, can be used. It consists of a series of microinjections in the top layers of the skin, which allows for slower drug dispersion than deep administration.

Mesotherapy is a minimally invasive approach that involves multiple dermal punctures to deliver tiny quantities of medicines or other bioactive substances through local intradermal therapy (LIT), where the injection location matches the region affected by the pathological condition. Modulating drug kinetics with longer local pharmacological activity, drug-sparing effects, a decreased risk of systemic interaction, and possible synergy with other treatments are just a few of the benefits of this method.

Three primary mechanisms of action appear to be involved in mesotherapy:

- The local action of the active ingredients,
- The mechanical distention of nearby tissues and sensitive fibers caused by the injected liquid and
- The reflex-based endorphin generation was induced by the introduction of needles.

E. M. AlEdani (✉)
Basra Medical College, Basrah, Iraq

E. M. AlEdani, H. Maibach (eds.), *Mesotherapy and Its Medical Applications*, Updates in Clinical Dermatology, https://doi.org/10.1007/978-3-031-76070-9_4

Myalgia, gout, headaches, neuralgia, low back pain, sports injuries, and musculoskeletal discomfort may all be effectively treated with mesotherapy.

Mesotherapy can be useful when systemic drugs are not tolerated and to synergize with other therapies.

4.1.2 *Mesotherapy Procedure*

Mesotherapy is a procedure that involves several "microinjections"of medication or active ingredients into the dermis via tiny needles. The angle at which the needle is inserted depends on the thickness of the skin. A single needle that is positioned between 30 and 45° from the surface of the skin, measuring 4 mm (27 gauge) or 13 mm (30 or 32 gauge), is used. Typically, 2 or 3 cm separates the injection sites, and 0.10–0.20 mL of product is used. The medicine can be diluted to treat larger areas, but this lowers the dosage, necessitating further or more frequent injections. After injection, the medication gradually penetrates the underlying tissues, reaching concentrations greater than those that are attained via intramuscular delivery (Fig. 4.1).

4.1.3 *Mesotherapy Treatment Benefits*

- This strategy is especially good for older people, those taking many medications, and those with diseases such as high blood pressure and gastrointestinal difficulties.
- Compared with oral or injectable drugs, mesotherapy allows for effective treatment with considerably lower doses.

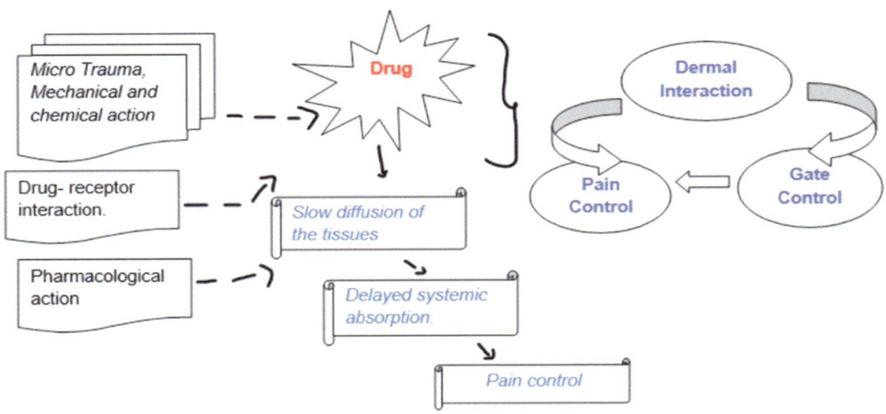

Fig. 4.1 Mesotherapy mode of action in the control of pain

- This ensures an optimal medication concentration at the target location.

4.1.4 Pain

According to the International Association for the Study of Pain, pain is "an unpleasant sensory and emotional experience associated with actual or potential tissue damage." Most scientists have different theories on how pain manifests. For example, Aristotle defined pain as a passion of the soul and thought that the heart was the source or center of pain processing. The ideas of neuroreceptors, nociceptors, and sensory input were postulated by Mueller, Van Frey, and Goldscheider in the nineteenth century.

In adults, the yearly incidence of moderate to severe back pain ranges from 10% to 15%, with a point prevalence ranging from 15% to 30%. According to estimates from the National Institute for Occupational Safety and Health, the annual cost of low back pain alone is between $50 billion and $100 billion per year.

4.1.4.1 Various Classifications of Pain

1. According to the recommendation, source, location, and duration (Fig. 4.2)
2. Predicted on Transmission (Fig. 4.3)

Because the analgesic response and pathophysiological causes vary, there is heterogeneity in the form of pain. There are no trustworthy objective indicators of pain, and physiologic signs and symptoms may coexist with pain. Multidimensional and rating scales are useful tools for evaluating the intensity of pain. Diverse approaches to treatment are needed because of the wide range of types of pain and how they

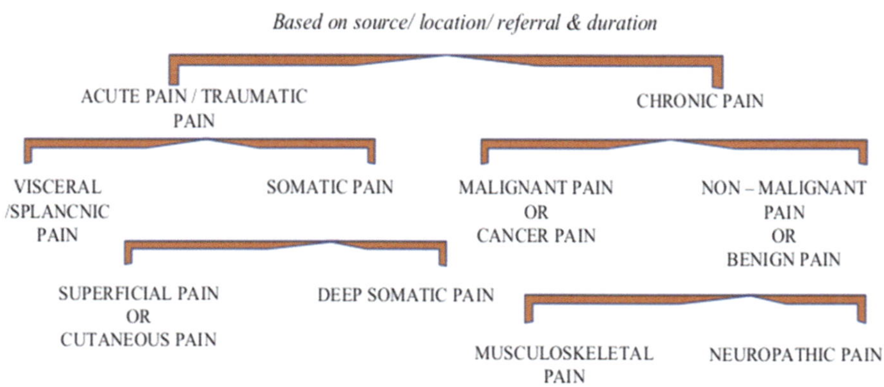

Fig. 4.2 Classification based on source/location/referral and duration

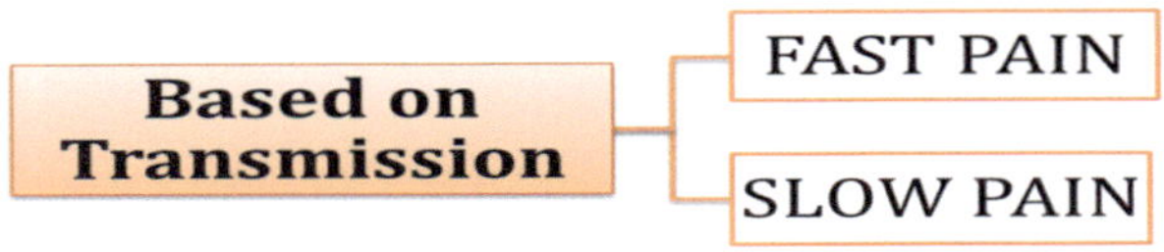

Fig. 4.3 Classification based on transmission

react to analgesic medications. A number of studies have shown that individuals with various musculoskeletal or posttraumatic diseases experience reduced pain.

In regard to the pharmacological treatment of acute pain, the systemic use of nonsteroidal anti-inflammatory medications (NSAIDs) is the first option. Owing to the high rate of NSAID side effects, including gastrointestinal toxicity, renal impairment, cardiovascular problems, and the possibility of drug–drug interactions, patients with cancer or those experiencing postoperative pain may need to supplement with an opioid analgesic. Mesotherapy is another treatment option for certain types of pain.

4.1.5 Connection Between Various Kinds of Pain and the Mesotherapy Approach

Since its initial development in 1952 as a pain relief technique, mesotherapy has been applied for a variety of aesthetic and medical goals. *Michel Pistor,* a French physician, invented mesotherapy 50 years ago. He used it as a unique analgesic therapy for a range of rheumatologic illnesses. Research has shown that compared with baseline, mesotherapy can effectively reduce pain for illnesses, including tendinopathy, back and cervical discomfort, and other musculoskeletal problems, by at least 50%. The goal of the treatment is to address the mesoderm, or middle layer of skin, and is thought to address underlying problems that lead to skin damage and discomfort, such as inadequate circulation and inflammation. It has been investigated as a potential therapy for a number of pain conditions, but its main application is in cosmetic medicine for fat reduction and skin renewal.

4.1.5.1 Acute Pain

Acute pain may be a useful physiological process for warning individuals of disease states and potentially harmful situations. Unfortunately, severe, unremitting, undertreated, acute pain, when it outlives its biological usefulness, can produce many deleterious effects (e.g., psychological problems). In normal scenarios, acute pain subsides quickly as the healing process decreases the pain-producing stimuli; however, in some instances, pain persists for months to years, leading to a chronic pain state with features quite different from those of acute pain.

Patients who are receiving anti-inflammatory therapy with NSAIDs (ketoprofen) and corticosteroids (methylprednisolone, MP), which are administered either via the mesotherapy technique or via the oral/intramuscular route, according to their pain score. Self-rated pain intensity was assessed via the VAS (0 = no pain, 100 = intolerable pain), a horizontal, unmarked 100 mm scale widely validated to assess pain.

Recent studies have shown for the first time that the administration of NSAIDs and corticosteroids via the mesotherapy technique can provide the same therapeutic benefit as conventional (oral and intramuscular) drug administration. Indeed, both treatments significantly reduced pain intensity and disability in daily life activities, and the effect was maintained for up to 6 months. These results are in accordance with previous studies showing that naproxen and diclofenac, which are administered via mesotherapy, are more effective than oral administration.

4.1.5.2 Chronic Pain

Severe psychological issues caused by dread and memories of previous pain might arise in people with chronic pain.

Chronic pain can be distinguished into four subtypes:

1. Pain that lasts longer than a typical recovery period following an acute injury;
2. Pain connected with a chronic illness;
3. Pain without a known organic cause; and
4. Pain involves both acute and chronic pain linked to cancer.

Chronic pain sufferers may develop analgesic dependency and tolerance, have difficulty sleeping, and are more sensitive to ecological changes that might exacerbate the pain response. Differentiating between acute and long-term discomfort is crucial for effective treatment approaches.

Therefore, in a holistic strategy for pain reduction, pharmaceutical therapy and psychological treatments work best when coupled with surgical techniques, anesthetic processes, and extra care measures. Some chronic pain patients report side effects from systemic therapy, whereas others have medical conditions that prevent them from using long-term medications. NSAIDs are frequently contraindicated or cannot be used for an extended period of time due to harmful cardiovascular or renal illness.

These factors make it simple to strike a balance between the chance of negative reactions and clinical safety when determining the lowest effective and highest tolerable dosage. Therefore, we discuss the impact of mesotherapy, which can work in concert with alternative treatments to control pain while lowering the necessary dosage and frequency of administration of some analgesics. Mesotherapy is not well supported when used alone to treat radicular pain or prolonged low back pain; injectable NSAIDs are recommended for treating persistent low back pain. Certain elements need to be taken into consideration when performing mesotherapy. Specific informed permission is needed, especially after the benefits and drawbacks of mesotherapy are outlined.

According to some studies, mesotherapy combined with the injection of lidocaine via superficial trigger points is a safe, efficient short-term treatment option for cerebral palsy.

Patients with traumatic diseases, acute myositis, tendinitis, lumbar discomfort, and shoulder-hand syndrome have been reported in some studies. After three mesotherapy injections spaced 3 days apart, vasodilators, NSAIDs, myorelaxants, and procaine were shown to alleviate pain in 83.6% of patients according to visual scales.

When NSAIDs are administered via mesotherapy, the therapeutic benefit outweighs that of oral medication delivery. In addition to receiving smaller dosages and infrequent dosing schedules, patients receiving mesotherapy also receive these drugs. Mesotherapy was administered with ease and speed, was well tolerated, and did not cause any allergic or local responses. Mesotherapy appears to represent an alternative therapeutic approach, particularly in the presence of acute, chronic diseases or comorbidities where there is a high risk of drug interaction or polypharmacy or when the use of conventional (oral or parenteral) NSAIDs is contraindicated. These benefits make mesotherapy a valuable technique for the management of painful musculoskeletal diseases.

When alternative treatments are unavailable, ineffective, or unfeasible for any other reason, mesotherapy may offer therapeutic advantages.

4.2 Mesotherapy and the Musculoskeletal System

4.2.1 Musculoskeletal System

In the musculoskeletal system, mesotherapy is occasionally used to treat pain and inflammation caused by conditions such as tendinitis, osteoarthritis, fibromyalgia, and muscular strains. Medication injections containing anti-inflammatories, analgesics, vitamins, minerals, and homeopathic treatments are sometimes used in mesotherapy sessions. Mesotherapy has been demonstrated to be more effective than systemic therapy in relieving local pain and functional limits caused by a variety of musculoskeletal illnesses.

Mesotherapy is used to treat musculoskeletal issues since it is a more focused and possibly more successful form of treatment than oral medications or other forms of therapy because these substances are injected directly into the affected region. To fully understand the benefits and risks of mesotherapy in this context, more studies are necessary, as the evidence for its effectiveness in treating musculoskeletal problems is still sparse.

4.2.1.1 Different Types of Musculoskeletal Pain According to Severity (Fig. 4.4)

Musculoskeletal system pain is divided into two categories, acute pain and chronic pain, depending on the intensity of the pain. Acute pain can be distinguished from actual and prospective tissue injury as an alert sensation. More than three months of chronic pain can be experienced, which is a significant and occasionally dangerous intensity (Fig. 4.5).

Pathological alterations in the musculoskeletal system can indicate a variety of acute and chronic illnesses, such as osteoarthritis, arthralgia, fibromyalgia, tunnel carpal syndrome, and other conditions that can be treated or managed with medicine. The mesotherapy treatment protocol was slightly modified on the basis of the situation, but the effectiveness remained the same.

4.2.2 Mesotherapy Treatment for Different Musculoskeletal System Illness Conditions

4.2.2.1 Osteoartritis

Among the degenerative illnesses of the musculoskeletal system, osteoarthritis (OA) is rather widespread. Joint degeneration, impaired cartilaginous tissue regeneration, and bone remodeling through chondral and synovial secondary responses are several types of joint injury that manifest as osteoarthritis (OA). As a first-line therapy for moderate osteoarthritis of the knee, acetaminophen/paracetamol has historically been the most commonly utilized painkiller. Compared with nonsteroidal anti-inflammatory medicines (NSAIDs), this medication seems to be less effective for moderate to severe symptoms. For the care of locoregional illnesses, mesotherapy offers an alternative therapeutic approach, especially in terms of pain control. Synergistic effects can result from the combination of mesotherapy and systemic treatment.

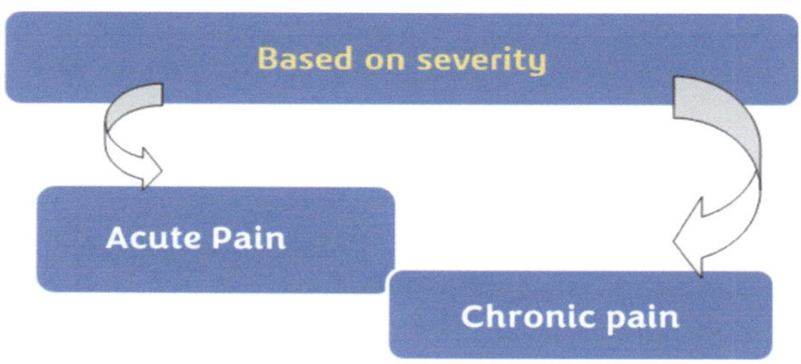

Fig. 4.4 Classification based on severity

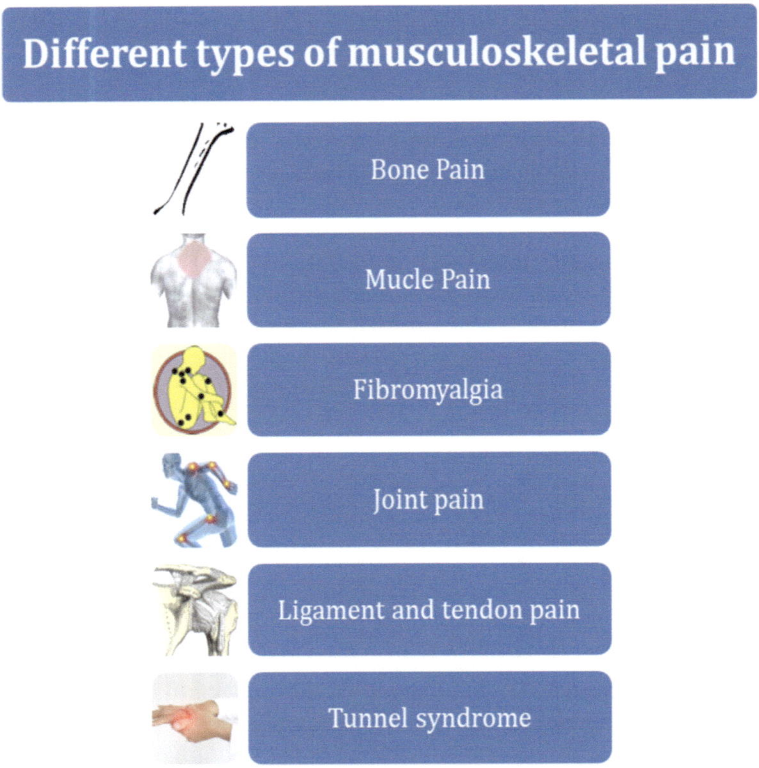

Fig. 4.5 Classification based on pathological changes

4.2.2.1.1 Treatment Procedure

Mesotherapy is a procedure that involves many "microinjections" of medication or active ingredients into the dermis via tiny needles. The angle at which the needle is inserted depends on the thickness of the skin. We advise the use of a single needle that is positioned between 30 and 45° from the surface of the skin, measuring 4 mm (27 gauge) or 13 mm (30 or 32 gauge). Generally, injection locations are spaced 2 or 3 cm apart, and 0.10–0.20 mL of product is utilized. The medication can be diluted to treat larger regions, but doing so lowers the dose and necessitates more or more frequent injections. After injection, the medication gradually penetrates the underlying tissues, reaching concentrations greater than those that are attained via intramuscular delivery. The medication exhibits varying pharmacokinetic properties (absorption, distribution, metabolism, and excretion) on the basis of the mode of administration.

Several studies have indicated that meshotherapy can be used to treat musculoskeletal pain issues in many patients, and most of these patients experience quick pain reduction, usually within the first three sessions. Six specific sites around the knee were subjected to mesotherapy via various protocols on the basis of whether the OA was in its acute or chronic phase. The results were compared across 3 months of oral diclofenac treatment. The patients' clinical states improved with both treatments, although mesotherapy had fewer adverse effects and was more effective in terms of WOMAC scores.

4.2.2.2 Fibromyalgia

The second most common rheumatological problem after osteoarthritis is fibromyalgia, a musculoskeletal ailment with an unclear cause that is more common in people between the ages of 20 and 50. There is a clear genetic predisposition at the root of the complex etiology of fibromyalgia, according to theory.

The hypothalamic–pituitary axis, neurotransmitter release abnormalities, hypersensitivity of the central nervous system, proinflammatory cytokine release, and imbalance between oxidizing and antioxidizing chemicals are all potential causes.

Broad-based chronic pain that resembles neuropathic pain in terms of neuropharmacology, physiopathology, and clinical presentation is one of the primary clinical presentations of fibromyalgia. In addition to asthenia, morning stiffness, sleep problems, paresthesia, headache, anxiety, melancholy, irritable bowel syndrome, Raynaud's phenomenon, and menstruation discomfort, the afflicted muscles, skin, ligaments, and tendons are frequently accompanied by allodynia and hyperalgesia.

The current multidisciplinary, gradual approach to treating fibromyalgia includes lifestyle and behavioral modifications, medication (such as antidepressants, muscle relaxants, and anticonvulsants), and nonpharmacological (such as exercise, relaxing massage therapy, connective massage, and electrotherapy, among others) treatments. An increasingly popular method that shows promise as a treatment option for fibromyalgia sufferers is antalgic mesotherapy.

4.2.2.2.1 Protocol for Mesotherapy Treatment

A skilled and qualified medical professional administered the mesotherapy via a 10 mL syringe fitted with sterile disposable needles with sizes of 4 and 6 mm. A pharmacological mixture of 2 mL (50 mg) of diclofenac, 2 mL (2 mg) of thiocolchicoside, and 1 mL (10 mg) of mepivacaine was created at every treatment session. Four milliliters of sodium chloride solution was then added. The operator begins by using gauze soaked in chlorhexidine to disinfect the skin. The disinfectant was applied, and it was permitted to work for 5 min. To avoid generating papules, 0.1–0.2 cc of this pharmacological mixture was given at each injection site, spaced approximately 2 cm apart, and injected at a depth of 1–3 mm. Following the injections, the patient's skin was cleaned once more, a covering patch was put on, and they were monitored for approximately 10 min while any potential negative reactions were noted. To avoid wetting the injection site for the next 12 h, patients were instructed.

The severity of fibromyalgia pain can be measured via the Fibromyalgia Impact Questionnaire (FIQ). The type of therapy used varied depending on severity. In addition, medical and nonmedical interventions alone are less effective as opposed to using a mix of mesotherapy techniques.

In the short term, mesotherapeutic treatment with diclofenac and thiocolchicoside has been shown to be superior to a placebo in terms of pain reduction, functional recovery, and quality of life. It has also been shown to be a safe and effective procedure for managing cervicalgia in fibromyalgia patients. Fibromyalgia may be regarded as a first-line treatment method. To evaluate their usefulness over time, further research is obviously still needed.

In light of some research, the majority of patients in Europe who have musculoskeletal pain are treated with nonpharmacological treatments, including exercise, physiotherapy, acupuncture, and herbal remedies, as their first-line treatment, followed by nonsteroidal anti-inflammatory medicines (NSAIDs).

4.3 Mesotherapy and Cellulitis

4.3.1 Cellulitis

Cellulite, a zigzag and rough (crimson skin) look created by trapped fat cells, is common in women, particularly in the hip, leg, abdomen, and arm areas. Cellulite, which is thought to be created only by the hormone estrogen, a woman-specific hormone, affects 85% of women today, while it is uncommon in men.

Cellulitis mesotherapy is a highly successful form of cellular treatment. Mesotherapy is a treatment for middle skin. Drugs given via ingestion or intravenously into the body do not reach enough quantities in the affected tissue and may cause systemic adverse effects. Mesotherapy is a method that involves administering tiny injections to the affected location.

4.3.2 Mesotherapy Treatment Process and Duration

The number of injections administered during treatment varies according to the size of the region to be treated, the condition, and the location. The pain is not severe. The amount of drug injected into the bloodstream is virtually minimal. It involves injecting 0.02–0.05 mL of medication solution transverse to the skin (4 mm deep) at approximately 1–2 cm intervals. Mostly used for fat reduction. The minor redness upon treatment, as well as the resulting bruises, are only transient.

The duration of therapy varies with the degree of cellulite. In general, it takes 2–3 sessions to observe effects. In most cases, 10 curative sessions are adequate once a week. However, cellulite mesotherapy, when combined with a healthy diet and regular exercise, can help minimize or eliminate detrimental behaviors.

4.3.3 Mesotherapy Without Needles

It is a novel method of mesotherapy that allows both ionized and neutral medicines to be delivered into the dermis and subcutaneous tissue. In this procedure, the targeted region is initially pretreated with dual-wavelength laser light, followed by four components:

- Electroporation is the process of producing electropores of 40–250 μm in size on the skin via electric waves at three distinct frequencies. The desired compounds are then made to pass through these pores via electro repulsion. However, the structure of the pores allows neutral substances to flow through.
- Active current: enhances vascularity, ensuring that an adequate amount of product reaches the location.
- Hydrophoresis occurs when water-soluble compounds enter the skin.
- Cryophoresis is the process by which freezing temperatures trap objects inside skin cells.

Mesotherapy without a needle (MWN) is primarily used to treat cellulite, but it is also useful for skin rejuvenation, hyperpigmentation of photoaging, wrinkle and pore reduction, and skin lifting. Compared with mesotherapy,

The MWN has the following advantages:

(a) no discomfort,
(b) no bruising, erythema, or swelling,
(c) materials can enter deeper levels,
(d) immediate/rapid reaction, and
(e) cost effectiveness.

4.4 Mesotherapy and Gingival Hyperpigmentation

4.4.1 Gingival Hyperpigmentation

One of the disorders in dermatology is hyperpigmentation. Skin color changes, discolorations, or darkening are its defining characteristics. The major cause of hyperpigmentation is the body's increased melanin concentration. Treatment for conditions that cause excessive pigmentation (melasma, sunspots, postinflammatory hyperpigmentation, mouth hyperpigmentation, etc.) requires long-term care and yields good outcomes despite low patient compliance. Oral formulations of therapeutic agents, including tranexamic acid, melatonin, and cysteamine hydrochloride, are used after topical formulations of traditional agents, such as hydroquinone, kojic acid, and glycolic acid, as first-line therapies for hyperpigmentation. Chemical peels and laser treatment administered under the supervision of qualified specialists are examples of second-line methods. Unfortunately, these treatments have drawbacks and side effects, including erythema, peeling skin, and drying out of the skin, and they take a long time. A common treatment for uneven skin tone and hyperpigmentation is mesotherapy. The unique combination of vitamins, antioxidants, and other nutrients used for injection works to reduce excess melanin and balance the color and texture of the skin.

Gingival hyperpigmentation, or mouth hyperpigmentation, is a hyperpigmentation syndrome. The gingiva line, the outer surface of the periodontium, extends to encompass the coronal section of the alveolar process and marks the boundary with the nonkeratinized buccal mucosa. Although the concepts, methods, and management of issues related to gingival melanin pigmentation are still being developed, melanin pigmentation frequently arises in the gingiva due to aberrant deposition of melanin, resulting in a black appearance in gums.

Different treatment techniques have been used to treat gingival hyperpigmentation conditions. These treatment techniques are called gingival depigmentation techniques (shown in Fig. 4.6).

This chapter mainly discusses how mesotherapy techniques work in the context of gingival hyperpigmentation. Before mesotherapy treatment, the level of gingival hyperpigmentation should be assessed via the melanin pigmentation index. Based on the scoring system

- Score 0: There is no pigment.

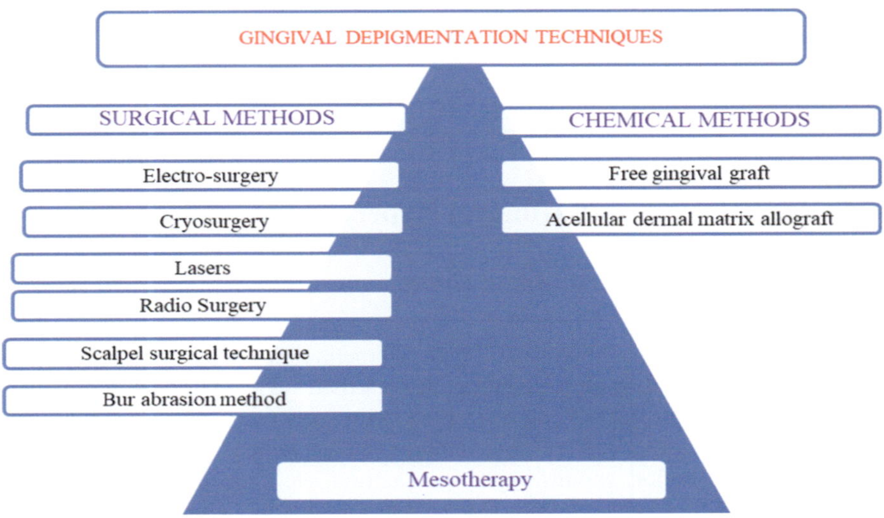

Fig. 4.6 Gingival depigmentation techniques

- Score of 1: One or more single pigmentation units in the papillary gingiva without any extension between adjacent solitary units;
- Score 2: Creation of an uninterrupted ribbon that branches out from nearby isolated units.

The method of mesotherapy is frequently used to establish different substances to address mouth hyperpigmentation. The primary foundation for the mesotherapy injection technique is the anatomical, histological, and geometric landmarks of the target tissues.

4.4.2 Mesotherapy Treatment Process (Fig. 4.7)

4.4.2.1 Pretreatment Instructions

- Caution should be taken in the presence of certain vitamins 3 days before the procedure (particularly ginkgo biloba and vitamin E).
- Disprin, Ecosprin, or aspirin was not used 3 days before the procedure.
- It is advisable to use an anesthetic gel 2 h before treatment to reduce discomfort.

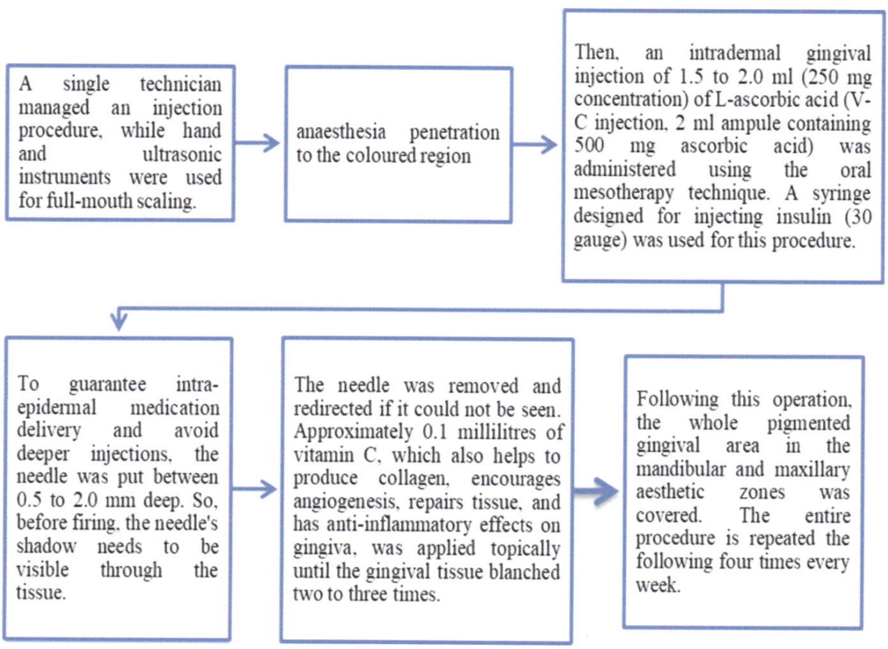

Fig. 4.7 Mesotherapy treatment process

4.4.2.2 Posttreatment Instructions

- There was no recovery period needed after mesh therapy.
- If a patient feels any discomfort, anti-inflammatory medicines can be used, as advised.
- Patients may experience burning and/or discomfort for 20 min after treatment.
- There may be some bruising in the treated area, resulting in some swelling in the treated area after 48 h.

Fewer studies have demonstrated that mesotherapy with vitamin C injections is far safer, more successful, and noninvasive than other gingival depigmentation treatments.

4.5 Mesotherapy and Burns

4.5.1 Burns

Burns and injuries are relatively connected and lead to a life and death situation. Although the skin is the main organ that is damaged, problems can emerge in multiple organs and systems. According to a survey, burns are the fourth most common form of injury worldwide, ranking after accidents while driving, tumbles and assault.

4.5.1.1 Classification of Burns

The burn etiologies include flames, chemicals (acids and/or alkalis), high and low electric voltages (>1000 mV, <200 mV), etc. Due to burn depth, burn depths are divided into 3°. It is shown in Fig. 4.8.

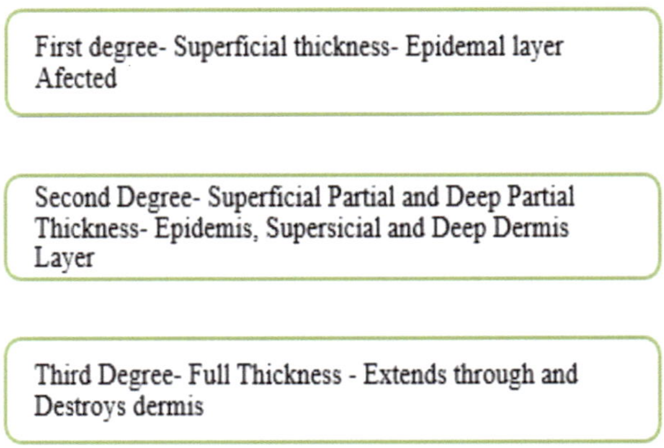

Fig. 4.8 Classification of Burns on the basis of degree of depth

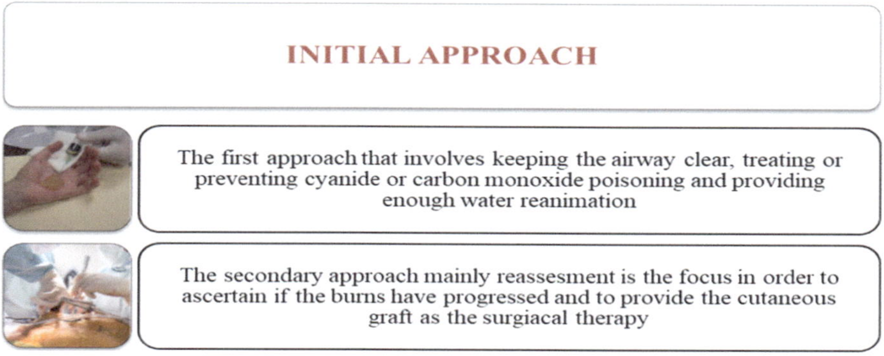

Fig. 4.9 Initial treatment approach for burns

The degree of burn treatment is different. The initial treatment for the burns is explained in Fig. 4.9. Surgical procedures are necessary for the management of full-thickness burn wounds to prevent them from worsening. Burn wound advancement can be avoided by being aware of the pathophysiologic underpinnings of burn wound conversion and by identifying signs of cutaneous burn damage.

4.5.2 Mesotherapy Process (Fig. 4.10)

4.6 Mesotherapy and Infections

4.6.1 Mesotherapy-Associated Nontuberculous Mycobacterial Infections

South American women of reproductive age were the most prone to nontuberculous mycobacterial skin infections caused by mesotherapy injections. Mesotherapy injections cause the skin to sores on the hips, thighs, belly, and buttocks. Women often target "problem areas", such as cellulite and gynoid fat, which can be challenging to eradicate with natural lifestyle changes. Infected skin lesions, whether nodules or abscesses, typically appear at several locations rather than as isolated or single lesions. This study suggests that infections are typically induced by contaminated mesotherapy fluid rather than bacterial infiltration through a skin barrier break.

Antibiotics are effective in treating most illnesses, although some patients need numerous courses of therapy. Infections take many months to cure and often result in scarring after treatment. These data indicate that mesotherapy-associated NTM

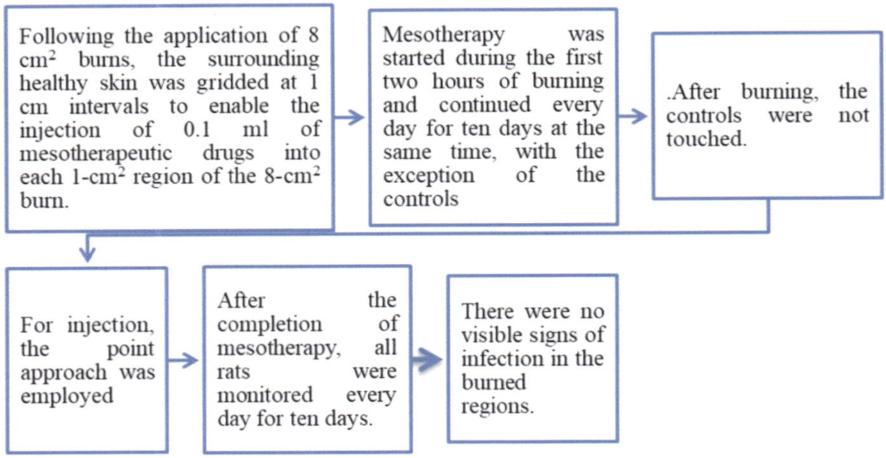

Fig. 4.10 Treatment process of burn mesotherapy

infections are challenging to cure and can lead to cutaneous complications that undermine the intended goal of enhancing the ability of the skin to look.

M. chelonae and M. abscessus are prevalent infections that might be resistant to medicines, making treatment challenging. Patients seeking mesotherapy should be aware that if a skin infection occurs as a result of surgery, they may need to take several antibiotics for months and may experience scarring.

There is no assurance of settlement. Many reported cases involved nonmedical or unconventional therapies, suggesting that these settings may be more vulnerable to contamination and consequences. Patients who receive mesotherapy injections outside of authorized healthcare settings are at greater risk and may not be aware of it.

Further Reading

1. Brauneis S, Araimo F, Rossi M, Russo D, Mammucari M, Maggiori E, di Marzo R, Vellucci R, Gori F, Bifarini B, Chiné E, Carpenedo R, Paolucci T, Giorgio C, Ritarossi R, Calò A, Luongo L, Natoli S. The role of mesotherapy in the management of spinal pain. A randomized controlled study. Clin Ter. 2023;174(4):336–42. https://doi.org/10.7417/CT.2023.2447.
2. Akbas I, Kocak AO, Kocak MB, Cakir Z. Comparison of intradermal mesotherapy with systemic therapy in the treatment of low back pain: a prospective randomized study. Am J Emerg Med. 2020;38(7):1431–5. Epub 2019 Dec 9. https://doi.org/10.1016/j.ajem.2019.11.044.
3. Carvalho RM, Barreto TM, Weffort F, Machado CJ, Melo DF. Use of vibrating anesthetic device reduces the pain of mesotherapy injections: a randomized split-scalp study. J Cosmet Dermatol. 2021;20(2):425–8. Epub 2020 Jul 8. https://doi.org/10.1111/jocd.13554.
4. Paolucci T, Bellomo RG, Centra MA, Giannandrea N, Pezzi L, Saggini R. Mesotherapy in the treatment of musculoskeletal pain in rehabilitation: the state of the art. J Pain Res. 2019;12:2391–401. PMID: 31440078; PMCID: PMC6679691. https://doi.org/10.2147/JPR.S209610.

5. Ronconi G, Ferriero G, Nigito C, Foti C, Maccauro G, Ferrara PE. Efficacy of intradermal administration of diclofenac for the treatment of nonspecific chronic low back pain: results from a retrospective observational study. Eur J Phys Rehabil Med. 2019;55(4):472–9. Epub 2019 Feb 15. https://doi.org/10.23736/S1973-9087.19.05432-7.
6. Akbas I, Kocak MB, Kocak AO, Gur STA, Dogruyol S, Demir M, Cakir Z. Intradermal mesotherapy versus intravenous dexketoprofen for the treatment of migraine headache without aura: a randomized controlled trial. Ann Saudi Med. 2021;41(3):127–34. Epub 2021 Jun 1. PMID: 34085549; PMCID: PMC8176379. https://doi.org/10.5144/0256-4947.2021.127.
7. Mammucari M, Maggiori E, Lazzari M, Natoli S. Should the general practitioner consider mesotherapy (intradermal therapy) to manage localized pain? Pain Ther. 2016;5(1):123–6. Epub 2016 May 26. PMID: 27229350; PMCID: PMC4912973. https://doi.org/10.1007/s40122-016-0052-3.
8. Alves JC, Santos A, Jorge P, Lafuente P. A multiple-session mesotherapy protocol for the management of hip osteoarthritis in police working dogs. Am J Vet Res. 2022;84(1):ajvr.22.08.0132. https://doi.org/10.2460/ajvr.22.08.0132.
9. Alves J, Jorge P, Santos A. Comparison of two mesotherapy protocols in the management of back pain in police working dogs: a retrospective study. Top Companion Anim Med. 2021;43:100519. Epub 2021 Feb 4. https://doi.org/10.1016/j.tcam.2021.100519.
10. Conforti G, Capone L, Corra S. Intradermal therapy (mesotherapy) for the treatment of acute pain in carpal tunnel syndrome: a preliminary study. Korean J Pain. 2014;27(1):49–53. Epub 2013 Dec 31. PMID: 24478901; PMCID: PMC3903801. https://doi.org/10.3344/kjp.2014.27.1.49.
11. Costantino C, Marangio E, Coruzzi G. Mesotherapy versus systemic therapy in the treatment of acute low back pain: a randomized trial. Evid Based Complement Alternat Med. 2011;2011:317183. Epub 2010 Sep 1. PMID: 20953425; PMCID: PMC2952299. https://doi.org/10.1155/2011/317183.
12. Di Cesare A, Giombini A, Di Cesare M, Ripani M, Vulpiani MC, Saraceni VM. Comparison between the effects of trigger point mesotherapy versus acupuncture points mesotherapy in the treatment of chronic low back pain: a short term randomized controlled trial. Complement Ther Med. 2011;19(1):19–26. Epub 2010 Dec 15. https://doi.org/10.1016/j.ctim.2010.11.002.
13. Ferrara PE, Ronconi G, Viscito R, Pascuzzo R, Rosulescu E, Ljoka C, Maggi L, Ferriero G, Foti C. Efficacy of mesotherapy using drugs versus normal saline solution in chronic spinal pain: a retrospective study. Int J Rehabil Res. 2017;40(2):171–4. https://doi.org/10.1097/MRR.0000000000000214.
14. Agostini F, Attanasi C, Bernetti A, Mangone M, Paoloni M, Del Monte E, Mammucari M, Maggiori E, Russo D, Marzo RD, Migliore A, Paolucci T. Web axillary pain syndrome-literature evidence and novel rehabilitative suggestions: a narrative review. Int J Environ Res Public Health. 2021;18(19):10383. PMID: 34639683; PMCID: PMC8507961. https://doi.org/10.3390/ijerph181910383.
15. Saggini R, Di Stefano A, Dodaj I, Scarcello L, Bellomo RG. Pes anserine bursitis in symptomatic osteoarthritis patients: a mesotherapy treatment study. J Altern Complement Med. 2015;21(8):480–4. Epub 2015 Jun 17. PMID: 26083769; PMCID: PMC4522948. https://doi.org/10.1089/acm.2015.0007.
16. Alves JC, Santos AM. Evaluation of the effect of mesotherapy in the management of osteoarthritis-related pain in a police working dog using the canine brief pain inventory. Top Companion Anim Med. 2017;32(1):41–3. Epub 2017 Jul 5. https://doi.org/10.1053/j.tcam.2017.07.002.
17. Babacan T, Onat AM, Pehlivan Y, Comez G, Tutar E. A case of the Behcet's disease diagnosed by the panniculits after mesotherapy. Rheumatol Int. 2010;30(12):1657–9. Epub 2010 Apr 17. https://doi.org/10.1007/s00296-009-1123-0.
18. Scaturro D, Vitagliani F, Signa G, Tomasello S, Tumminelli LG, Picelli A, Smania N, Letizia MG. Neck pain in fibromyalgia: treatment with exercise and mesotherapy. Biomedicine.

2023;11(3):892. PMID: 36979871; PMCID: PMC10045341. https://doi.org/10.3390/biomedicines11030892.
19. Chen L, Li D, Zhong J, Qiu B, Wu X. Therapeutic effectiveness and safety of mesotherapy in patients with osteoarthritis of the knee. Evid Based Complement Alternat Med. 2018;2018:6513049. Erratum in: Evid Based Complement Alternat Med 2018 May 14;2018:5327589. doi: 10.1155/2018/5327589. PMID: 29507592; PMCID: PMC5817326. https://doi.org/10.1155/2018/6513049.
20. Alves JC, Santos A, Jorge P, Lafuente P. Multiple session mesotherapy for management of coxofemoral osteoarthritis pain in 10 working dogs: a case series. Can Vet J. 2022;63(6):597–602. PMID: 35656532; PMCID: PMC9112366.
21. Mammucari M, Gatti A, Maggiori S, Sabato AF. Role of mesotherapy in musculoskeletal pain: opinions from the Italian Society of Mesotherapy. Evid Based Complement Alternat Med. 2012;2012:436959. Epub 2012 May 13. PMID: 22654954; PMCID: PMC3359685. https://doi.org/10.1155/2012/436959.
22. Farpour HR, Estakhri F, Zakeri M, Parvin R. Efficacy of Piroxicam mesotherapy in treatment of knee osteoarthritis: a randomized clinical trial. Evid Based Complement Alternat Med. 2020;2020:6940741. PMID: 32831875; PMCID: PMC7421712. https://doi.org/10.1155/2020/6940741.
23. Tseveendorj N, Sindel D, Arman S, Sen EI. Efficacy of mesotherapy for pain, function and quality of life in patients with mild and moderate knee osteoarthritis: a randomized controlled trial. J Musculoskelet Neuronal Interact. 2023;23(1):52–60. PMID: 36856100; PMCID: PMC9976173.
24. Faetani L, Ghizzoni D, Ammendolia A, Costantino C. Safety and efficacy of mesotherapy in musculoskeletal disorders: a systematic review of randomized controlled trials with meta-analysis. J Rehabil Med. 2021;53(4):jrm00182. PMID: 33764479; PMCID: PMC8814845. https://doi.org/10.2340/16501977-2817.
25. Kocak AO. Intradermal mesotherapy versus systemic therapy in the treatment of musculoskeletal pain: a prospective randomized study. Am J Emerg Med. 2019;37(11):2061–5. Epub 2019 Feb 28. https://doi.org/10.1016/j.ajem.2019.02.042.
26. Caruso MK, Roberts AT, Bissoon L, Self KS, Guillot TS, Greenway FL. An evaluation of mesotherapy solutions for inducing lipolysis and treating cellulite. J Plast Reconstr Aesthet Surg. 2008;61(11):1321–4. Epub 2007 Oct 22. https://doi.org/10.1016/j.bjps.2007.03.039.
27. Rosato L, Lazzeri D, Campana M, Vaccaro M, Campa A, Ciappi S, Nisi G, Brandi C, Grimaldi L, D'Aniello C. Mesotherapy should not replace the surgical approach in the treatment of benign symmetric lipomatosis. Aesthetic Plast Surg. 2011;35(2):278–80. https://doi.org/10.1007/s00266-010-9571-1.
28. Sylwia M, Krzysztof MR. Efficacy of intradermal mesotherapy in cellulite reduction—conventional and high-frequency ultrasound monitoring results. J Cosmet Laser Ther. 2017;19(6):320–4. Epub 2017 Jun 7. https://doi.org/10.1080/14764172.2017.1334927.
29. Vannucchi G, Campi I, Covelli D, Forzenigo L, Beck-Peccoz P, Salvi M. Treatment of pretibial myxedema with dexamethazone injected subcutaneously by mesotherapy needles. Thyroid. 2013;23(5):626–32. https://doi.org/10.1089/thy.2012.0429.
30. Esmat SA, El-Sayed NM, Fahmy RA. Vitamin C mesotherapy versus diode laser for the esthetic management of physiologic gingival hyperpigmentation: a randomized clinical trial. BMC Oral Health. 2023;23(1):899. PMID: 37990224; PMCID: PMC10662509. https://doi.org/10.1186/s12903-023-03614-7.
31. El-Mofty M, Elkot S, Ghoneim A, Yossri D, Ezzatt OM. Vitamin C mesotherapy versus topical application for gingival hyperpigmentation: a clinical and histopathological study. Clin Oral Investig. 2021;25(12):6881–9. Epub 2021 May 8. Erratum in: Clin Oral Investig. 2021 Dec;25(12):6891. doi: 10.1007/s00784-021-04110-4. https://doi.org/10.1007/s00784-021-03978-6.

32. Buz A, Görgülü T, Olgun A, Kargi E. Efficacy of glutathione mesotherapy in burns: an experimental study. Eur J Trauma Emerg Surg. 2016;42(6):775–83. Epub 2015 Nov 27. https://doi.org/10.1007/s00068-015-0607-8.
33. Singsing ME, Duncan SG, Vachon MJ, Goff HW. Clinical features of mesotherapy-associated nontuberculous mycobacterial infections: a systematic review. Int J Womens Dermatol. 2022;8(4):e059. https://doi.org/10.1097/JW9.0000000000000059.

Chapter 5
Toxicology and Sides Effects of Mesotherapy

Esraa M. AlEdani and Hagar Elgezeri

5.1 Hair Loss at Injection Sites for Mesotherapy

Mesotherapy has been used as a treatment for hair loss; paradoxically, hair loss at injection sites has been reported as a side effect. There are different compositions of mesotherapy, with patients being unaware of what is being injected into their scalp. Some mesotherapy formulations, such as minoxidil, include plant extracts, vitamins and drugs with known effects on hair growth. Regardless of the different formulations used, some patients present with different types of hair loss, which is often associated with erythema, edema and pain on the scalp skin.

A 42-year-old patient developed frontal fibrosing alopecia 3 months after receiving mesotherapy treatment for her severe migraine headache. The cocktail contained a beta blocker [propranolol], which has been associated with the induction of lichenoid skin reactions. The patient received 4 sessions of mesotherapy for her severe migraine headache. The patient underwent a session every 15 days, and it included bilateral injections within the deep dermal region (4 mm), which were separated by 2 cm along the frontal line and in the eyebrows. After treatment, the patient experienced trichodynia as well as paresthesia after the injections, followed by slight recession of the frontal hair line. Upon examination, the skin was devoid of hair follicular opening with recession of the hair line, which was then confirmed by a trichoscope showing rarefaction of hair follicles, absence of vellus hair, perifollicular erythema and hyperkeratosis. Biopsy was performed, and the findings were consistent with frontal fibrosing alopecia.

E. M. AlEdani (✉)
Basra Medical College, Basrah, Iraq

H. Elgezeri
Faculty of Medicine, Cairo University, Giza, Egypt

E. M. AlEdani, H. Maibach (eds.), *Mesotherapy and Its Medical Applications*, Updates in Clinical Dermatology, https://doi.org/10.1007/978-3-031-76070-9_5

However, the etiology of frontal fibrosing alopecia has not been fully clarified. Some factors have been postulated to play a role, such as hormones, genetics, immune dysfunction and environmental factors. However, the patient without the aforementioned risk factors developed frontal fibrosing alopecia 3 months after her mesotherapy treatment.

The other 2 patients developed acute patchy alopecia after receiving mesotherapy for androgenetic alopecia. The first patient was a 32-year-old patient who presented with inflammatory irregular patches of alopecia on the right parietal scalp a few days after a mesotherapy session with a cocktail that contained a heparinoid derivative mesoglycan [prisma]. Upon examination, an 8-cm long and 2- to 3-cm wide erythematous bald patch associated with edema was noted. Biopsy confirmed a decrease in hair density with the absence of terminal anagen hair follicles. The second patient was a 22-year-old woman who presented with multiple patches of alopecia after 4 sessions of mesotherapy sessions that involved homoeopathic agents. Upon examination, the patient presented 3 round erythematous patches of alopecia from 2 to 4 cm long and 2 to 3 cm wide. The patches had some remaining hairs. Biopsy revealed a significant decrease in hair density with increased telogen germinal units and catagen follicles.

Finally, a case series presented 3 more patients who developed patchy hair loss at injection sites for mesotherapy for scalp alopecia. The first patient was a 30-year-old patient who presented with 5 circumscribed tender patches of hair loss on her frontal scalp after 5 sessions of mesotherapy with a cocktail including 2 mL dutasteride 0.0005%, a mixture of growth factors, multivitamins, amino acids and minerals. Development of the lesions took place 1 week after her last session. The lesion was accompanied by pain, which led her to discount the treatment. Similar to previous cases, the lesions were clinically devoid of hair. On dermoscopy, multiple white dots with a marked decrease in follicular openings were observed along with perifollicular and interfollicular mild scaling and several vellus hairs. The second patient was a 29-year-old patient who presented with a single erythematous, tender and crusted plaque associated with decreased hair density on the frontal scalp after 1 year of monthly mesotherapy treatment with the same cocktail as the aforementioned patient. The dermoscopic findings were similar to those of the previous case. Finally, a 34-year-old patient developed 2 linear erythematous atrophic scars devoid of hair after receiving her 3rd mesotherapy session of an unknown mesotherapy cocktail. Her dermoscopic findings were also quite similar to previous findings: erythema along with white patches, mild perifollicular and interfollicular scaling, white dots, several vellus hairs and arborizing capillaries along with decreased follicular opening. Biopsy was then performed, and the histological findings revealed a normal epidermis with a marked reduction in the number of hair follicles and increased thickening of collagen along with mild perifollicular and perivascular lymphohistocytic infiltrates.

Although the cocktails used in the previous patients were different and the patients' presentations were not identical, a significant decrease in the number of hair follicles was observed among all patients, which should raise some concerns about the use of mesotherapy as a treatment for hair loss.

5.2 Arthrosis

Mesotherapy with acetyl-L-carnitine (ALC) has been marketed for weight reduction, as it enhances and boosts fat metabolism by facilitating the transportation of long-chain fatty acids across the mitochondrial membrane as well as their esterification. However, given that ALC has immunomodulating effects, it is worth mentioning that a case in which a 31-year-old woman—with no family history of systemic lupus erythematosus (SLE) or other autoimmune disorders—developed systemic lupus erythematosus a few weeks after mesotherapy injections with ALC for weight reduction. The treatment included intradermal injections in the abdominal region with a total of 50 mg of ALC. Although the treatment was performed to reduce her weight, no reduction in her weight was observed. Her SLE symptoms manifested first 2 weeks after treatment on the skin in the form of painful, red maculopapular lesions that were not responsive to oral antibiotics, and then her symptoms continued to escalate to fever, arthralgia, tiredness, malar rash, headache, oliguria, and pleuritic chest pain and continued to worsen until she was hospitalized 2 months after her symptoms started. During her hospitalization, she showed some nervous manifestations characterized by generalized seizures. Initially, she was given treatment to control her condition, which needed to be mostly controlled, but she suffered from renal insufficiency that led to glomerulosclerosis.

5.3 Abdominal Hematoma

Common and minor mesotherapy side effects include small, easily resorbed hematomas at the injection areas, but a more serious and less reported side effect following mesotherapy is a large abdominal hematoma. A case report presented a 50-year-old woman who developed gastrointestinal manifestations such as epigastric pain, nausea, vomiting and abdominal tumefaction 2 months after undergoing mesotherapy for abdominal wall obesity. The treatment modality included 11 applications of siliceous and vegetal extracts. Her symptoms persisted for 7 months. Endoscopy revealed a 6-cm heterogeneous mass compressing the anterior gastric wall. On CT scan, the mass appeared as a solid mass compressing the gastric wall and the transverse colon with infiltration of the mesenteric structures. Owing to the suspicion of sarcoma, further investigations, including total colonoscopy and exploratory laparotomy, revealed an outcome that was suggestive of sarcoma. Then, subtotal gastrectomy with gastrojejunal anastomosis was performed. The pathological findings were then consistent with an organized hematoma without evidence of any malignant features. Importantly, the patient had no previous history of bleeding disorders or trauma, which leaves us with the probability of a link between the mesotherapy injections and the establishment of the hematoma.

5.4 Edema

Mostly, milder side effects may be associated with mesotherapy, but more serious side effects of mesotherapy therapy have been reported, namely, angioedema. For example, with one of the most common forms of hair loss, androgenetic alopecia, topical minoxidil, has been approved as a treatment for both women and men, as well as as an oral finasteride for men. To enhance the results, mesotherapy cocktails have also been used along with the aforementioned treatments for, perhaps, a better outcome.

In a case series, 14 patients experienced frontal edema after receiving mesotherapy injections for androgenetic alopecia. The treatment modality included intradermal injections of mesotherapy cocktails, including minoxidil, finasteride, growth factors, panthenol, biotin and steroids. To clarify the treatment modality further, 10 of the 14 patients received dutasteride with 2 mL of lidocaine every 3 months. The other 4 patients received a mixture containing minoxidil or finasteride with or without panthenol and biotin injected monthly. The edema mostly presented in the first 2 sessions and typically lasted from 1 to 4 days and subsided with cold compression. The majority of patients, 8 out of 14, experienced edema after the first session, which lasted mostly for 1 to 7 patients, constituting 50% of the patients. The presentation of edema was frontal for most of the patients, but 2 patients presented with orbital edema, and another patient presented with lateral edema. In all of these cases, lidocaine was the anesthetic used, which may have caused edema. Other ingredients of mesotherapy, such as minoxidil and dutasteride, may play a role.

In another case report, a 45-year-old female patient with androgenetic alopecia presented with perioribital edema along with erythema on the forehead 24 h after her first mesotherapy session. The cocktail used in her mesotherapy treatment included dutasteride. The patient then received patch testing for solutions with dutasteride in alcohol at the following concentrations: 0.001%, 0.01% and 0.05% and 20% propylene glycol. She showed positive reactions to dutasteride and propylene glycol. This finding shows that angioedema is, in fact, a presentation of allergic contact dermatitis.

While the aforementioned case reports report edema following mesotherapy injections, it is important to mention that the solutions used in both are different. This leaves us unsure of the exact mechanism behind the formation of angioedema. It is important to investigate whether the ingredients being injected, namely, minoxidil, dutasteride or lidocaine, are possibly triggers for angioedema or if the technique itself and the volume of substances being injected may predispose patients to frontal edema.

5.5 Psoriasis

A patient with psoriasis for 10 years received mesotherapy with a cocktail of aminophilline, xantinol nicotinate and lidocaine for the treatment of neuralgic sciatica on her left side. Two weeks later, at the injection site on her left thigh, she started developing circular psoriatic lesions along with worsening of preexisting lesions on other parts of the body, such as the scalp, trunk and limbs. Additionally, pustular lesions also developed on the palms and soles. While other factors may trigger psoriasis, clinical and laboratory examination findings excluded other trigger factors for psoriasis in this patient. This response may be due to the trauma caused by mesotherapy needle injections as well as the substances that are injected, especially in patients with unstable psoriasis.

5.6 Delirium with Psychosis

Despite the common side effects of mesotherapy, a case report of a 40-year-old woman who experienced delirium associated with psychotic features was reported after her first mesotherapy treatment, with an estimated duration of 8–12 h. The mesotherapy treatment consisted of bilateral injection of both thighs of unknown content that the patient was not aware of. She was brought to the emergency department in a state of confusion and distress with abnormal speech. She was then treated with an intramuscular injection of haloperidol (5 mg), and her symptoms resolved, resulting in a calm and oriented state. Importantly, the patient was not on any medications that could contribute to her delirium, and she had no personal or family history of psychiatric disorders. Later, extensive work-up revealed findings that were all within normal ranges. She was then admitted to the psychiatry inpatient service. After 2 days of close observation with no administration of medications, she was discharged with no residual symptoms.

5.7 Skin Ulcers

5.7.1 Facial Cutaneous Ulcers

A 26-year-old Saudi female experienced skin eruption on her left cheek for 2 weeks. The eruption occurred 2 weeks after mesotherapy MT injections in the same locations. The patient was informed that the injectable was used to "whiten and smooth''the skin and was only administered on the left side of the face. However, the actual substance of the injectable remains unknown. Examination revealed numerous slightly sensitive 0.5-cm ulcerated nodules with erythematous borders on the left cheek. There is no option for collection or discharge. Outside cultures collected by the treating physician were reported to be negative. The patient was prescribed 100 mg of doxycycline daily and 2% fucidic acid +1% hydrocortisone acetate cream twice daily for ulcers. At the 1-week follow-up, all ulcers had healed, with erythematous hypertrophic scars. We were unable to obtain the ingredients of the injected material from the treating physician. The patient was informed that it included "vitamins".

5.7.2 Noninfectious Granulomatous Panniculitis

A 37-year-old Caucasian woman was referred for consultation after a 5-month history of panniculitis in her buttocks and lower extremities, which corresponded to the areas of prior mesotherapy injections for "cellulite." Six months before presentation, the patient received three mesotherapy injections at a licensed practical nurse's home office. The patient indicated that the injection fluid contained deoxycholate. After the injections, the patient had "lumps" beneath her skin that grew, were sensitive and red, discharged yellow fluid, and eventually healed, leaving scars behind. The patient acquired lesions in all regions treated with mesotherapy injections. Examination of the buttocks, thighs, knees, and lower legs revealed many violaceous sensitive nodules with and without crusted erosions, as well as hyperpigmented macules. She denied having systemic symptoms. Repeated biopsies revealed deep dermal and pannicular inflammation, as well as granulomatous inflammation with fibrosis. The microbial strains were negative. The results from direct immunofluorescence investigations were negative. Tissue cultures for bacteria, mycobacteria, fungi, and viruses yielded no microorganisms across three occasions. Polarization and X-ray tissue examination did not reveal any foreign material. Amylase and lipase levels were normal, and no evidence of alpha1-antitrypsin insufficiency was detected. A diagnosis of mesotherapy-induced noninfective scarring occurred as a result of granulomatous panniculitis.

Previous therapies included oral trimethoprim, sulfamethoxazole, clindamycin, levofloxacin cephalexin and topical mupirocin without improvement; she showed slight improvement after a course of oral prednisone. After several months of dapsone therapy at 100 mg per day, the creation of new lesions slowed, and dapsone therapy ultimately stopped. Her scarring is substantial and has been linked to psychological discomfort.

5.7.3 Cutaneous Granulomatous Reaction

A 28-year-old woman was referred for many sores on her belly and legs. She underwent three sessions of mesotherapy using a combination of procaine, silica (organic silica), and buflomedil for body contouring. The sessions were conducted by a beautician at a private facility. Two weeks following the previous treatment, few red pruritic papules appeared at the application locations, stretching from the belly and legs to the thighs. Her personal and familial background was unimpressive. Dermatologic examination revealed red pruritic papules and nodules on the patient's belly and legs. Histopathology revealed hyperkeratosis, acanthosis, and degradation of dermal collagen. Epithelioid histiocytes accumulated in a palisading pattern surrounding the necrotic regions. Large lymphocytic cells were also observed. A cutaneous granulomatous response to mesotherapy was identified. Biochemical parameters, including blood glucose and thyroid hormones, were within normal ranges. After 4 months of systemic corticosteroid use (oral deflazacort, 60 mg/day), there was no improvement. Dapsone (100 mg/day) was administered. The lesions improved significantly after 1 month; however, the patient was not followed up further.

5.7.4 Granuloma Annulare

A 34-year-old Caucasian woman with Fitzpatrick Skin Type II and Type I diabetes mellitus reported persistent red spots on her abdomen 2 to 3 weeks after receiving mesotherapy injections from a nondermatologist at a Colorado medical resort. She has experienced sporadic red spots on her shins for years. The patient came 7 months after receiving mesotherapy injections to dissolve fat in her belly. The differential diagnosis of granuloma annulare includes necrobiosis lipoidica diabeticorum and a cutaneous foreign body response. Histological confirmation of granuloma annulare was obtained with a 4-mm punch biopsy of one plaque. Treatment via intralesional steroid injections was planned.

5.7.5 Subcutaneous Nodules

A 27-year-old woman underwent seven sessions of mesotherapy (5% DW [dextrose] 8 cc 1 lidocaine 2 cc) once or twice a week to minimize cellulite in her abdomen. One month following the initial injection, she presented with painful erythematous nodules in the belly. After 1 month, several nodules spontaneously developed ulcers with yellowish serous discharge.

She came to our department 4 months after the first session. Skin examination revealed four erythematous and painful subcutaneous lumps on her belly. A biopsy of one lesion revealed chronic panniculitis, including fat necrosis, thrombosis in small- and medium-sized arteries, and lipomembranous alterations. A culture of the biopsy samples was negative for fungi, bacteria, and mycobacteria. Laboratory examinations, including a full blood count and chemical tests, revealed no abnormalities. There was no substantial medical history or family history. Treatment for panniculitis included an intralesional injection of 2.5 mg/mL triamcinolone acetonide, as well as oral administration of minocycline (100 mg/day for 2 weeks) and prednisolone (20 mg/day for 2 weeks), which resulted in a minor improvement. After 4 weeks, the nodules exhibited liquefaction, fat necrosis, ulceration, and yellowish serous discharge. After 2 weeks of dressing and topical administration of mupirocin ointment, the lesions progressively healed with scarring.

Further Reading

1. Frioui R, Mokni S, Tabka M, Belajouza C, Denguezli M. Frontal fibrosing alopecia following beta blocker injectable mesotherapy: is it more than a simple coincidence? Dermatol Ther. 2022;35(1):e15206. Epub 2021 Dec 1. https://doi.org/10.1111/dth.15206.
2. Duque-Estrada B, Vincenzi C, Misciali C, Tosti A. Alopecia secondary to mesotherapy. J Am Acad Dermatol. 2009;61(4):707–9. Epub 2009 Jul 3. https://doi.org/10.1016/j.jaad.2008.11.896.
3. El-Komy M, Hassan A, Tawdy A, Solimon M, Hady MA. Hair loss at injection sites of mesotherapy for alopecia. J Cosmet Dermatol. 2017;16(4):e28–30. Epub 2017 Feb 3. https://doi.org/10.1111/jocd.12320.
4. Colón-Soto M, Peredo RA, Vilá LM. Systemic lupus erythematosus after mesotherapy with acetyl-L-carnitine. J Clin Rheumatol. 2006;12(5):261–2. https://doi.org/10.1097/01.rhu.0000239831.84504.0b.
5. Gamo R, Aguilar A, Cuétara M, Gonzalez-Valle O, Houmani M, Martín L, Gallego MA. Sporotrichosis following mesotherapy for arthrosis. Acta Derm Venereol. 2007;87(5):430–1. https://doi.org/10.2340/00015555-0271.
6. Brandão C, Fernandes N, Mesquita N, Dinis-Ribeiro M, Silva R, Lomba Viana H, Moreira DL. Abdominal hematoma—a mesotherapy complication. Acta Derm Venereol. 2005;85(5):446. https://doi.org/10.1080/00015550510027829.
7. Melo DF, Saceda-Corralo D, Tosti A, Weffort F, Carla Jorge M, de Barros CC, de Melo CR, Starace M. Frontal edema due to mesotherapy for androgenetic alopecia: a case series. Dermatol Ther. 2022;35(2):e15247. Epub 2021 Dec 13. https://doi.org/10.1111/dth.15247.
8. Magdaleno-Tapial J, Valenzuela-Oñate C, García-Legaz-Martínez M, Martínez-Domenech Á, Alonso-Carpio M, Talamantes CS, Zaragoza-Ninet MG, Zaragoza-Ninet V. Angioedema-like contact dermatitis caused by mesotherapy with dutasteride. Contact Dermatitis. 2020;83(3):246–7. Epub 2020 Jul 1. https://doi.org/10.1111/cod.13585.
9. Onder M, Atahan CACA, Oztaş P, Oztaş MO. Temporary henna tattoo reactions in children. Int J Dermatol. 2001;40(9):577–9. https://doi.org/10.1046/j.1365-4362.2001.01248.x.
10. Tor PC, Lee TS. Delirium with psychotic features possibly associated with mesotherapy. Psychosomatics. 2008;49(3):273–4. https://doi.org/10.1176/appi.psy.49.3.273.
11. Al-Khenaizan S. Facial cutaneous ulcers following mesotherapy. Dermatol Surg. 2008;34(6):832–4; discussion 834–5. Epub 2008 Mar 31. https://doi.org/10.1111/j.1524-4725.2008.34155.x.
12. Davis MD, Wright TI, Shehan JM. A complication of mesotherapy: noninfectious granulomatous panniculitis. Arch Dermatol. 2008;144(6):808–9. https://doi.org/10.1001/archderm.144.6.808.
13. Gokdemir G, Küçükünal A, Sakiz D. Cutaneous granulomatous reaction from mesotherapy. Dermatol Surg. 2009;35(2):291–3. https://doi.org/10.1111/j.1524-4725.2008.01053.x.
14. Lee DP, Chang SE. Subcutaneous nodules showing fat necrosis owing to mesotherapy. Dermatol Surg. 2005;31(2):250–1. https://doi.org/10.1097/00042728-200502000-00027.
15. Strahan JE, Cohen JL, Chorny JA. Granuloma annulare as a complication of mesotherapy: a case report. Dermatol Surg. 2008;34(6):836–8. Epub 2008 Mar 31. https://doi.org/10.1111/j.1524-4725.2008.34156.x.

Chapter 6
Mesotherapy as a Lucrative Business

Amr Elrosasy and Esraa M. AlEdani

6.1 Introduction to the Mesotherapy Market

Mesotherapy has emerged as a promising market globally, with tremendous growth from $158.83 million in 2022 to a projected value of $846.41 million by 2028. A remarkable annual growth rate of 32.16% during the forecast period was a notable addition to the mesotherapy market. Mesotherapy has received unprecedented attention and acclaim in recent years from a separate treatment to an increasing segment in the broader landscape of the industry, with factors such as increasing consumer demand for beauty options instead of implants, the growing number of dermatological problems and medical technological advances.

At its core, mesotherapy encompasses fundamental changes in improving skin tone and rejuvenation, providing a holistic approach to address a wide range of skin issues. This approach requires active ingredients customized with vitamins, minerals, amino acids and pharmaceuticals that penetrate the mesodermal layer of skin. The product serves a wide range of purposes, from skin rejuvenation and hydration to the reduction of fine lines, wrinkles and hyperpigmentation.

The appeal of mesotherapy lies in its multifaceted benefits, addressing a variety of skin care needs and concerns. In addition to combating signs of aging, dealing with wrinkles, or rejuvenating tired and dull skin, mesotherapy offers a versatile solution that meets skin-seeking consumer requirements and, because mesotherapy is less damaging and has a shorter recovery time, positions itself as the preferred option for individuals seeking cosmetic rehabilitation without the inherent risks and downtime associated with traditional surgery.

A. Elrosasy (✉)
Faculty of Medicine, Cairo University, Giza, Egypt

E. M. AlEdani
Basra Medical College, Basrah, Iraq

E. M. AlEdani, H. Maibach (eds.), *Mesotherapy and Its Medical Applications*, Updates in Clinical Dermatology, https://doi.org/10.1007/978-3-031-76070-9_6

With the growing demand for mesotherapy treatments, the market has seen innovative products and technologies designed to improve treatment effectiveness and patient outcomes.

Advanced delivery systems to sophisticated devices and supportive therapies.

As mesotherapy continues to gain mainstream traction and acceptance, it is poised to revolutionize the aesthetic dermatology landscape by offering a more robust alternative to traditional skin care techniques but with caution, taking into consideration the regulatory environment, safety considerations and the ethical requirements of mesotherapy's rapid rise through a collaborative ecosystem of health professionals, developers including manufacturers, regulators and consumers. The mesotherapy market can continue to thrive and grow, opening new frontiers in skin care and beauty enhancement.

6.2 Impact of the COVID-19 Pandemic

However, the COVID-19 pandemic has also affected the mesotherapy market. As the virus mesotherapy has spread around the world, causing health and economic problems, and the market faces many challenges. Aggressive product launches, program option cancellations and supply chain disruptions slowed market growth. Consumer interest in mesotherapy products and services has decreased due to uncertainty and economic instability.

Despite these challenges, however, there are signs of recovery. As the economy recovers and the healthcare industry returns to normal, the mesotherapy market is expected to grow further.

People still want skincare solutions, driven by a growing awareness of overall wellness and a desire to look younger. In addition, the rise of telemedicine and virtual counseling has made mesotherapy accessible, breaking down geographical barriers and expanding the market.

6.3 Key Players and Market Dynamics

The mesotherapy market consists of a variety of companies, from big brand names to small start-ups, all of which are trying to succeed in the growing skin care industry. The leader of this group is Koru Pharmaceuticals Co., which is the largest brand in the country. Ltd., Meso Fusion, Percebel, Tuscany Cosmetics, Demoaroma, Plural, Mesoessence, Companies such as Galderma Laboratories L.P., Revitacare, Mesoaesthetic, and DERMEDICS International. These companies are highly influential due to their strong research and development capabilities, strategic networks, and broad markets.

Innovation is a key factor in shaping the mesotherapy market. Companies invest heavily in research and development to make treatments safer and more effective.

New formulations and delivery methods have been developed, and cutting-edge technology has been used to push the boundaries of skin care.

Competition in the mesotherapy market is fierce, with companies fighting for market share through aggressive marketing, unique products and partnerships. Differentiation matters, and companies are working hard to offer specialty treatments, targeted treatments, or better customer experiences.

Regionally, the mesotherapy market varies considerably. North America leads the way with its robust research infrastructure, growing customer base and good regulations. Europe has a long history of new skincare, whereas Asia Pacific, the Americas and Latin America offer attractive growth opportunities as their markets mature.

Despite the potential for growth, companies face challenges. Compliance is tricky, and safety is a major concern. Companies need to rigorously test and monitor their products once they reach the market.

In summary, the mesotherapy market is competitive and constantly evolving, driven by innovation and changing consumer preferences. Companies need to stay adaptable and meet regulatory standards and customer demands. By fostering innovation and collaboration, they can succeed in this fast-paced industry and continue to grow and evolve.

6.4 Market Segmentation and Applications

The mesotherapy market can be segmented into different segments, including product types, applications, end-user segments, and regional variation. This classification helps us understand the different needs and preferences of consumers and stakeholders in the field of mesotherapy.

6.4.1 Product Types

Mesotherapy solutions involve different formulations, each designed to address specific skin problems and needs. These products generally contain a blend of vitamins, minerals, amino acids, and chemicals, carefully selected to nourish and rejuvenate the skin in addition to masks, potions, special tools and other products of interventions that improve treatment efficacy and outcomes.

6.4.2 Applications

Mesotherapy has many applications in dermatology and aesthetics, showing versatility and effectiveness. Some common uses are as follows:

1. Anti-aging: Mesotherapy helps reduce fine lines, wrinkles and skin aging stimulating collagen and elastin.
2. Young Face: Refreshes skin with a custom-made blend of ingredients that improves hydration and addresses dryness and uneven tone.
3. Hair restoration: Mesotherapy can stimulate hair growth and deliver nutrients directly to hair follicles.
4. Cellulite Reduction: Targets localized fat deposits and improves skin texture by breaking down fat cells and increasing lymphatic circulation.
5. Acne Treatment: Mesotherapy combats acne by addressing inflammation and improving sebaceous production.

6.4.3 End-User Segments

Mesotherapy services are used by various health professionals, beauty professionals and consumers. These include:

1. Hospitals and clinics: Primary providers of mesotherapy treatments, offering specialized services.
2. Beauty Centers and Medspas: They offer complete skin care solutions in a luxurious environment.
3. At-home devices: Customers can now use mesotherapy devices at home for professional results.

6.4.4 Regional Dynamics

Different regions have different levels of acceptance of and growth rates for mesotherapy. North America and Europe are leading the way in skincare innovation, and emerging markets in Asia Pacific, Latin America and the Middle East will soon embrace mesotherapy treatments. Each region presents unique opportunities and challenges on the basis of cultural factors and different laws or health care systems.

Overall, mesotherapy market segmentation helps us understand the diverse needs of customers and stakeholders. Using this information, companies can tailor their products, services and marketing strategies to meet the needs of specific audiences, driving growth and differentiation in a competitive marketplace.

6.5 Opportunities and Challenges

The mesotherapy market provides significant opportunities for innovation and growth but also poses challenges that need to be carefully considered. Understanding these developments is important for stakeholders aiming to maximize the potential of mesotherapy and effectively control the risks.

6.5.1 Opportunities

1. Growing demand for noninvasive cosmetic products: Mesotherapy offers a nonsurgical alternative and is attractive to consumers seeking safe and customizable treatment options with little rehabilitation time.
2. Advances in technology and drug development: Innovations in the design and supply chain improve the efficacy and safety of mesotherapy treatments.
3. Expanding the consumer base: Mesotherapy is gaining popularity among individuals from diverse backgrounds, reflecting a broader trend in skin care capability and availability.
4. Global market expansion: The adoption of mesotherapy is rapidly expanding in emerging markets in regions such as Asia Pacific and Latin America, opening new avenues for market growth and product diversification.

6.5.2 Challenges

1. Regulatory compliance and safety: Meeting stringent regulatory standards and ensuring product safety are ongoing challenges for mesotherapy companies.
2. Scientific credentials: Despite the popularity of mesotherapy, hard scientific evidence is lacking, making it difficult to gain acceptance among skeptics and regulators.
3. Market Concentration: Intense competition and market congestion make it difficult for firms to differentiate and market their niche.
4. Educational and training gaps: Addressing differences in physician training and education is important to ensure safe and effective delivery of mesotherapy treatments.

Stakeholders must invest in rigorous research to address these challenges effectively.

Standardization of protocols and collaboration with regulatory bodies. By doing so, they can increase the credibility and efficacy of mesotherapy while ensuring patient safety and satisfaction.

6.6 Cost and Financial Considerations

Mesotherapy treatments constitute a significant financial investment for patients, with session costs typically ranging from $200—$600 and patients typically needing approximately ten sessions. However, the economic implications extend beyond the upfront cost, including factors such as treatment efficacy, long-term outcomes, and cost-effectiveness considerations.

6.6.1 *Cost-Effectiveness and Treatment Efficacy*

While mesotherapy holds the promise of nonsurgical body contouring and skin rejuvenation, the variable efficacy of treatments introduces uncertainty into the cost-effectiveness equation.

Patients may undergo multiple sessions, each accompanied by substantial financial burdens, only to achieve suboptimal or inconsistent results. This disparity between cost and efficacy undermines the perceived value proposition of mesotherapy, fueling skepticism among patients as well as healthcare providers.

6.6.2 *Financial Investment Versus Treatment Outcomes*

The discrepancy between the high cost of mesotherapy treatments and the unpredictable nature of treatment outcomes underscores the complex interplay between financial considerations and patient expectations. Patients may be willing to invest significant financial resources in pursuit of aesthetic improvements, only to be disappointed by the lack of results or transient benefits of mesotherapy. This mismatch between financial investment and treatment outcomes further stimulates the disappointment and dissatisfaction of patients, contributing to the controversial nature of mesotherapy as a cosmetic procedure.

6.6.3 *Variable Efficacy and Patient Satisfaction*

The variable efficacy of mesotherapy treatments poses a challenge to patient satisfaction and loyalty. While some individuals may experience dramatic improvements in skin texture, tone, and contouring following mesotherapy, others may experience minimal benefit or encounter adverse effects. This heterogeneity in treatment outcomes highlights the importance of personalized treatment approaches, thorough patient counseling, and realistic expectation management to optimize patient satisfaction and reduce the risk of treatment-related regret.

6.6.4 Scientific Evidence and Regulatory Approval

The scarcity of scientific evidence and regulatory approval surrounding mesotherapy further complicates cost–benefit analysis for patients and healthcare providers. In the absence of robust clinical data and standardized treatment protocols, patients must weigh the potential risks and benefits of mesotherapy against alternative treatment modalities with a more established evidence base. Moreover, the lack of regulatory oversight raises concerns about patient safety, treatment efficacy, and practitioner accountability, increasing financial and ethical considerations associated with mesotherapy.

In conclusion, the cost and financial considerations surrounding mesotherapy treatments are many-sided, encompassing aspects such as treatment efficacy, patient satisfaction, and scientific evidence, and regulatory approval. While mesotherapy offers the allure of nonsurgical aesthetic enhancements, the high cost, in addition to the variable treatment outcomes, underscores the need for informed decision-making, evidence-based practice, and patient-centered care. By addressing these financial considerations in a transparent and holistic manner, stakeholders can foster greater trust, satisfaction, and value for patients seeking mesotherapy treatments.

6.7 Regulatory Landscape and Recommendations

Regulatory frameworks governing the delivery of mesotherapy treatments and permitted substances vary widely among different countries. In Brazil, for example, members have been known to administer injections in nonmedical settings, raising serious safety concerns.

Furthermore, pharmaceutical advertising often creates the misconception that mesotherapy is a treatment for a wide range of cosmetic and medical treatments. It is crucial for regulatory authorities to establish stringent regulations to safeguard patient safety and regulate the dissemination of mesotherapy treatments by unauthorized individuals.

6.8 Conclusion and Future Perspectives

In conclusion, mesotherapy presents an attractive opportunity within the cosmetic industry, with potentially significant economic benefits. Companies can participate in this lucrative market by addressing key challenges related to security, efficiency and compliance.

The global mesotherapy market is expected to reach USD 846.41 million by 2028, representing significant growth from USD 158.83 million in 2022. This growth trajectory highlights the enormous profit potential of companies operating in this area. To take advantage of this opportunity and maximize value, industries must prioritize scientific integrity and evidence-based practices.

Investing in research and development to prove the effectiveness and safety of mesotherapy treatments is essential to building consumer trust and loyalty. In addition, compliance with regulations is critical for businesses to reduce legal risk and gain confidence in the marketplace.

Innovation and differentiation are key success factors in the mesotherapy industry. Investing in Advanced technologies, adjunctive therapies and unique treatments can help businesses stand out in a competitive market and attract sophisticated consumers. Additionally, networking and Strategic collaboration can expand markets and unlock new revenue streams. By partnering with dermatologists, pharmacies, and other healthcare providers, companies can tap into diverse consumer groups to generate profits. Looking ahead, the future of mesotherapy as a profitable profession is bright.

Further Reading

1. Atiyeh BS, Ibrahim AE, Dibo SA. Cosmetic mesotherapy: between scientific evidence, science fiction, and lucrative business. Aesthetic Plast Surg. 2008;32:842–9.
2. Kandhari R, Kaur I, Sharma D. Mesococktails and mesoproducts in aesthetic dermatology. Dermatol Ther. 2020;33(6):e14218.
3. Atiyeh BS, Abou GO. An update on facial skin rejuvenation effectiveness of mesotherapy EBM V. J Craniofac Surg. 2021;32(6):2168–71.
4. Sylwia M, Krzysztof MR. Efficacy of intradermal mesotherapy in cellulite reduction–conventional and high-frequency ultrasound monitoring results. J Cosmet Laser Ther. 2017;19(6):320–4.
5. Global mesotherapy market size, share and industry analysis by regions, countries, types, and applications, forecast to 2028. https://www.360marketupdates.com/global-mesotherapy-market-24104371.

Index

E. M. AlEdani, H. Maibach (eds.), *Mesotherapy and Its Medical Applications*, Updates in Clinical Dermatology, https://doi.org/10.1007/978-3-031-76070-9

MIX
Papier aus verantwortungsvollen Quellen
Paper from responsible sources
FSC® C105338

If you have any concerns about our products,
you can contact us on
ProductSafety@springernature.com

In case Publisher is established outside the EU,
the EU authorized representative is:
Springer Nature Customer Service Center GmbH
Europaplatz 3, 69115 Heidelberg, Germany

Printed by Libri Plureos GmbH
in Hamburg, Germany